# Health Minutes

★★★★★

## Ginelle Edmondson, MPH, BSN, RN

Health Ministries Director
Mountain View Conference of Seventh-day Adventists

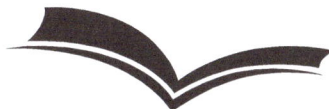

**TEACH Services, Inc.**
PUBLISHING
www.TEACHServices.com • (800) 367-1844

Copyright © 2022 Ginelle Edmondson

Copyright © 2022 TEACH Services, Inc.

ISBN-13: 978-1-4796-1476-9 (Paperback)

ISBN-13: 978-1-4796-1477-6 (ePub)

Library of Congress Control Number: 2022907027

**TEACH Services, Inc.**
P U B L I S H I N G
www.TEACHServices.com • (800) 367-1844

# Table of Contents

# CHAPTER 1

# 5 Essential Minerals[1]

Minerals are elements in our body. Although iron tends to be most well known, these five other minerals are also important.

Chromium. Chromium may be involved in fat metabolism, and it helps to control blood sugar in diabetics. Almonds are a good source.

Potassium. This mineral helps control blood pressure, muscle function, and nerve impulses. Potassium is excreted in sweat and can be replaced by sports drinks. It can also be found in bananas, citrus fruits, legumes, and nuts.

Magnesium. Magnesium reduces muscle cramps, strengthens bones, regulates heart rhythm, supports a healthy immune system and blood clotting. Studies have shown it may control blood sugar in diabetics. Magnesium is found in green vegetables such as lettuce, spinach, green beans, and peas.

Calcium. Calcium is essential for healthy bones, teeth, muscles, and the contraction of blood vessels. Good sources are broccoli, kale, and spinach.

Zinc. Zinc helps keep your immune system strong, aids in wound healing and in protein and DNA synthesis, and is essential for chemical reactions. Good sources of zinc include beans, fortified breakfast cereals, nuts, and whole grains. Good nutrition can supply all the daily mineral requirements.

---

[1] "The 5 Most Important Minerals You Should Be Getting In Your Diet," https://1ref.us/1sy accessed 12/6/20.

# CHAPTER 2

# 5 Reasons to Avoid Snacking[2]

*I praise you because I am fearfully and wonderfully made;*
*your works are wonderful, I know that full well.* (Psalm 139:14, NIV)

Even the most sophisticated computer can't match the "human machine" that God made. However, to maintain optimal performance we need to follow His instruction manual. By putting whatever tastes good into our bodies whenever we feel like it, we've become like grazing cows. Studies estimate that most people get about 30% of their food through snacking.

> *By putting whatever tastes good into our bodies whenever we feel like it, we've become like grazing cows.*

What's wrong with snacking? Dr. John A. Scharffenberg, health consultant to the General Conference of Seventh-day Adventists, gives five reasons not to snack:

1. Teeth are de-mineralized for two hours following a meal and then are remineralized. Continual eating interrupts this process and increases the risk of tooth decay.

2. Triglycerides (fats) increase when we eat. This increases the stickiness of the platelets and red blood cells. It may increase the risk of forming blood clots that could result in a heart attack.

3. Blood sugar levels increase when we eat, which requires insulin to process. Continual stimulation can cause excess levels of insulin which could increase the risk of heart attack.

4. Eating 2–3 large meals burns about 40 more calories per day than eating 6–8 smaller meals.

5. Grazing provokes more frequent gastric juice secretion, which may irritate ulcers.

Maybe it's time we return to the instruction manual! Ellen White wrote:

[2] Brittany Mullins, "Which is better? 3 meals a day vs 5-6 mini meals," updated June 6, 2019, available at https://1ref.us/1sz, accessed 12/6/20.

"Regularity in eating is very important for health of body and serenity of mind. Never should a morsel of food pass the lips between meals" (*Counsels on Health*, p. 118).

God's marvelous machine would function better if we followed His instruction manual and quit grazing like cattle.

# CHAPTER 3

# Eight Tips to Boost Energy Levels[3]

Don't have the energy to get things done? Try these eight ideas to feel more invigorated.

1. Plan Ahead.
2. Delegate. Feeling overwhelmed with too much to do? Ask for help.
3. Eat. Even children know that energy comes from food. However, bad eating habits, like skipping breakfast, signals your body to store fat, leaving you lethargic. Grabbing a sugary pastry is just as bad as no food at all.
4. Relax. Take 15–30 minutes today to do something to refresh your spirit.
5. Say, "NO." Decide what's important and say "no" to the rest.
6. Sleep. The pioneers slept 10 hours a night, but today the norm is less. The result is more frequent illness, feeling exhausted, and more accidents. Go to bed and wake up at the same time every day. Your body needs at least eight hours of sleep a night to see health benefits.
7. Stimulate your brain. Reduce boredom by trying an activity you are curious about or by enrolling in a class. Search for service opportunities.
8. Expand your horizons. Don't just read through these energy-boosting tips but make it a priority to try them. You'll have more energy to embrace life.

In one of her books on health, Ellen White wrote: "God has provided us with constitutional force, which will be needed at different periods of our life. If we recklessly exhaust this force by continual overtaxation, we shall sometimes be losers. Our usefulness will be lessened, if not our life itself destroyed" (*Christian Temperance and Bible Hygiene*, p. 64).

---

[3] "How To Get More Energy: 20 Tips To Boost Your Energy And Get More Done," available at https://1ref.us/1t0, accessed 12/5/20.

# CHAPTER 4

# Activated Charcoal[4]

The process of making charcoal is fairly simple. Once the water has evaporated with some volatile elements, the familiar black pieces are created. Nowadays, charcoal can be produced for medicinal use from animal bones or coal. Historically charcoal has come from plant-based sources such as hardwood, bamboo, coconut, or peat.

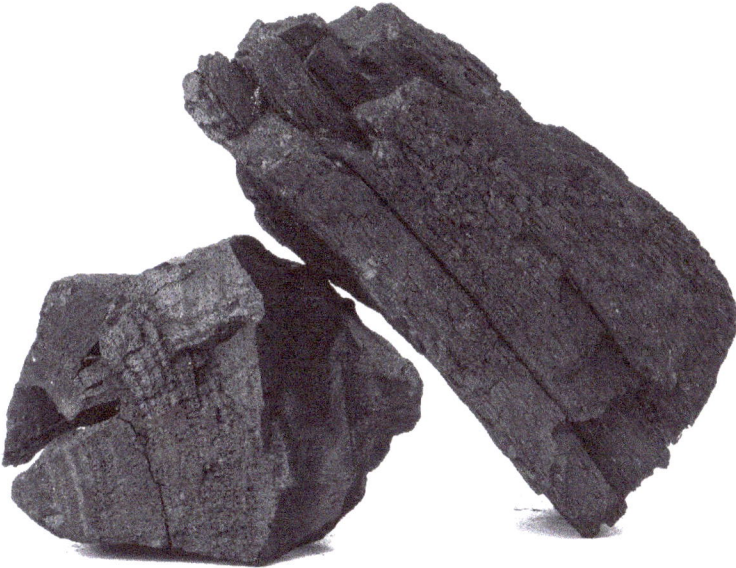

Activated charcoal has an incredible ability to adsorb, which is when atoms or molecules adhere to its irregular surface. Because activated charcoal is not processed, it remains in the gastrointestinal tract when it is ingested, and it eliminates toxins via a bowel movement. It is also effective against bad breath, gas, and intestinal disorders.

The action of adsorption should not be confused with absorption, which occurs when a substance passes into or through a tissue like liquid

[4] Jennifer Huizen, "What are the benefits of activated charcoal?" January 10, 2020, available at https://1ref.us/1t1, accessed 11/27/20.

in a sponge. Charcoal will only attach to substances inside the stomach or intestines. Once they have been absorbed by the GI tract, activated charcoal can no longer retrieve a toxin that has been ingested.

When charcoal is applied externally, the property of adsorption extracts toxins and inflammatory substances out of the body through the skin. It is best not to apply charcoal poultices onto open wounds, as a tattooing effect may occur.

Charcoal can be used for acne, arthritis, poisoning, burns, cholesterol, insect bites, ear infections, pain, odors, and much more.

The only known side effects are a sporadic irritation of the bowel in particular conditions and the prolongation of the transit time, that is, constipation.

# CHAPTER 5

# The Adventists' Health[5]

Adventists support the biblical diet of grains, nuts, and vegetables. They encourage a well-balanced diet that includes nuts, fruits, legumes (beans), and foods that are low in sugar, salt, and refined grains.

The Adventist diet prohibits foods deemed "unclean" by the Bible, such as pork and shellfish. The only endorsed beverage is water: 5 glasses a day to stay alive, 8 to feel great, and 10 to rejuvenate.

The first Adventist health study was the analysis of 34,000 individuals in California over the course of 14 years. The results revealed those who adhere to this routine lived about ten years longer than those who didn't.

Below are the five practices that were found to boost one's life expectancy.

1. Consuming a plant-based diet
2. Not smoking
3. Maintaining an average body weight
4. Eating a handful of nuts 5 times a week
5. Consistent physical exercise

These Adventists are Americans who live among us, drive by the same fast-food restaurants, shop at the same grocery stores, work at the same jobs, even go to the same church, and breathe the same air. Yet, they live a decade longer.

These folks could be the group that leads Americans back to the original diet just as God chose the Israelites to be a nation to point others toward Him.

---

[5] Aaron Gilbreath, "Why Do Seventh-Day Adventists Live Longer Than Most Americans?" available at https://1ref.us/1t2, accessed 12/5/20.

# CHAPTER 6

# The Avocado[6]

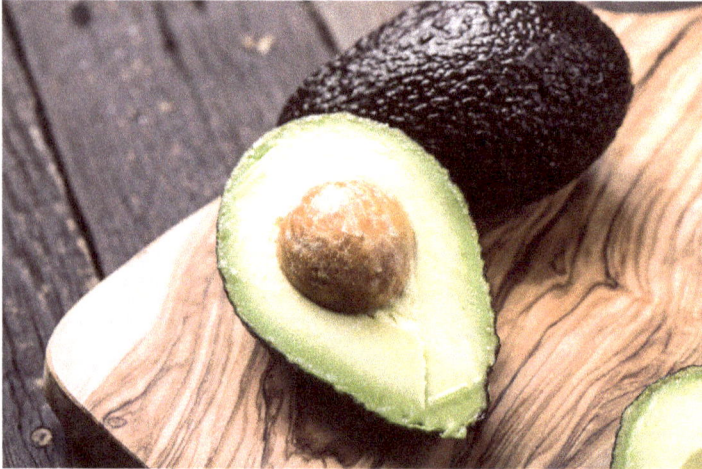

Native to Mexico and Central America, the avocado is a fruit that is often used in salads, and it is the main ingredient in guacamole.

Although the fat content of the avocado is high, the fats it contains are beneficial. Studies have shown that these fats can reduce levels of bad cholesterol and can reduce the risk of stroke and heart disease. In addition, participants in a study who consumed half an avocado with their lunch reported a 40% decrease in appetite for three hours after the meal.

> *Although the fat content of the avocado is high, the fats it contains are beneficial.*

An average avocado contains around four grams of protein, which is more than many other fruits.

Avocados are an excellent source of potassium, containing more per weight than bananas. Also avocados are rich in vitamin K, vitamin B9, vitamin B6, vitamin B5, vitamin C, and vitamin E.

---

[6] Ocean Robbins, "Everything You Need to Know About Avocados + 15 Science-Backed Reasons to Eat These Fabulous Fruits," published February 6, 2019, available at https://1ref.us/1t3, accessed 11/27/20.

If you're tired of eating beans to get your fiber, try some avocados. A medium avocado contains 11 grams of fiber, with 75 percent of it being insoluble (the form that speeds up the digesting process), and the other 25 percent being soluble (the form that is responsible for making you feel "full").

Other benefits associated with the fruit include lowering cholesterol levels, reducing the risk of diabetes, promoting lower body weight, and preventing cancer.

Forget butter, jam, mayonnaise, or peanut butter. Avocados make the best spread for bread. An avocado can also be used as a meat substitute in sandwiches and salads.

# CHAPTER 7

# Vitamin B12 is an Essential Nutrient[7]

Vitamin B12 is required for our DNA and cell division, red blood cells, and the protective layers around the nerves of the body.

Vitamin B12 is imperative for vegetarians since it is found only in animal-based products including red meats, poultry, seafood, dairy products, and eggs. However, there are plant-based foods that are fortified with the vitamin, such as ready-to-eat breakfast cereals, plant beverages made from soy, rice, almonds, coconut, oats, hazelnuts, or cashews, vegetarian meat, and nutritional yeast, such as Red Star®.

B12 can also be taken as a supplement and as part of many multivitamins. It is also present in spirulina, seaweed, and fermented foods, such as tempeh.

Those over 50 should get a significant amount of their dietary B12 from foods fortified with B12 or they should take a consistent supplement.

The General Conference Nutrition Council recommends that the total vegetarian should consume foods fortified with vitamin B12 or use a 500-$\mu$g supplement of vitamin B12 three to four times a week. Supplementation is vital for a pregnant or breast-feeding woman. The elderly, vegetarians, and lacto-ovo-vegetarians with decreasing consumption of dairy and eggs should have their vitamin B12 status checked at least on an annual basis.

---

[7] Team, General Conference Nutrition Council, "Vitamin B12 for the Vegetarian," available at https://1ref.us/1t4, accessed 8/3/21.

# CHAPTER 8

# Barley[8]

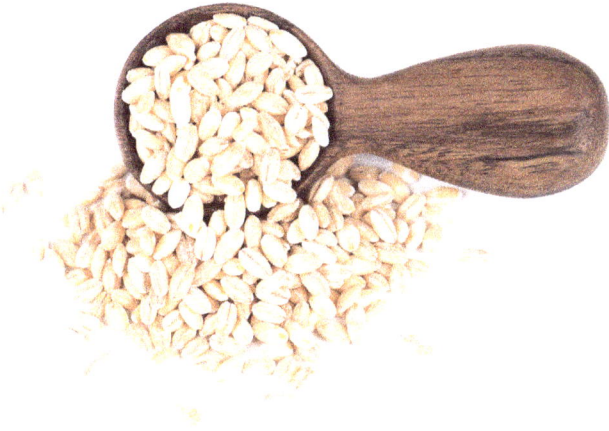

A versatile cereal grain with a rich nut-like flavor, barley has a chewy, paste-like consistency. It is often used in soups to boost the nutritional value, add thickness, or enhance the flavor. Some of the key nutrients found in barley include dietary fiber, selenium, tryptophan, copper, manganese, phosphorus, and niacin. All of these nutrients are beneficial to overall health.

In addition to bulk and decreasing the risk of colon cancer and hemorrhoids, barley's dietary fiber also provides food for the "good" bacteria found in the large intestine. These bacteria are thought to also be responsible for the cholesterol-lowering benefits of fiber. Barley's fiber can also prevent higher blood sugar levels and can prevent gallstones.

Barley has been found to have a much higher fiber content than do oats.

Other benefits from steady consumption of barley include cardiovascular benefits, prevention of heart failure, a lower risk of type 2 diabetes, protection against breast cancer, and defense against childhood asthma.

The nutritional benefits of barley can be reaped by mixing barley flour with wheat flour for baking, adding cracked barley or barley flakes to hot cereal, or pearled barley to your favorite stews and soups.

---

[8] Wholegrainscouncil.org, "Health Benefits Of Barley," available at https://1ref.us/1t5, accessed 12/1/20.

# CHAPTER 9

# The Benefits of Fasting[9]

Fasting is biblical. Fasting goes hand-in-hand with prayer. Many scriptures discuss fasting. For example, in Acts 13:2, as the early believers served the Lord and fasted, the Holy Ghost announced: "Separate me Barnabas and Saul for the work whereunto I have called them." Esther mentioned fasting in her instructions to Mordecai: "Go, gather together all the Jews that are present in Shushan, and fast ye for me, and neither eat nor drink three days, night or day: I also and my maidens will fast likewise; and so will I go in unto the king, which is not according to the law: and if I perish, I perish" (Esther 4:16).

What is fasting? It is abstaining from food or reducing food and drink intake every so often.

Since the body is unable to get its energy from food during fasting, it dips into glucose stored in the liver and muscles. This begins around eight hours after the last meal has been consumed. When the glucose has been expended, the body burns fat as a source of energy, which can result in weight loss.

As well as aiding weight loss, the use of fat for energy can preserve muscle and reduce cholesterol levels.

If someone has not fasted before, they should consider starting with a one-day fast to try it out and make sure there are no adverse effects.

## Tips

Fasting can be mentally and physically strenuous, so individuals should:

- Eat foods that are high in energy before fasting.
- Pick a time that will allow for rest, such as a day when you are not at work.
- Circumvent fasting if unwell or tired.
- Avoid demanding exercise.

[9] Natalie Butler, RD, LD, "All you need to know about water fasting," available at https://1ref.us/1t6, accessed 8/3/21.

Consider building up to a fast slowly, perhaps by reducing the size of your meals.

During a fast, it is essential to drink enough water throughout the day.

When ending a water fast, a person should not eat too much at once but should rather eat in increments to avoid a stomach ache or feeling sick.

Fasting deprives the body of the fuel it needs, so expect to feel a bit tired and low on energy. A lack of food can also make people feel dizzy, weak, or nauseous, and, if these symptoms are particularly bad, it is important to eat something.

Get plenty of rest. Sitting down and avoiding intense exercise can help conserve energy. It is common to feel irritable or tired, but seek medical advice if you feel disoriented while fasting.

# CHAPTER 10

# Benefits of Pure Air[10]

*Air, air, the precious boon of heaven, which all may have, will bless you with its invigorating influence. Welcome it, cultivate a love for it, and it will prove a precious soother of the nerves. The influence of pure, fresh air is to cause the blood to circulate healthfully through the system. It refreshes the body and renders it strong and healthy, while at the same time its influence is decidedly felt upon the mind, imparting a degree of composure and serenity. It excites the appetite, and renders the digestion of food more perfect, and induces sound and sweet sleep. (Testimonies for the Church, vol. 1, p. 702)*

> *Air, air, the precious boon of heaven, which all may have, will bless you with its invigorating influence.*

*Air must be in constant circulation to be kept pure. (Healthful Living, p. 71)*

*Sleeping rooms especially should be well ventilated, and the atmosphere made healthy by light and air. Blinds should be left open several hours each day, the curtains put aside, and the room thoroughly aired. (Spiritual Gifts, vol. 4a, p. 142)*

*The effects produced by living in close, ill-ventilated rooms are these: The system becomes weakened, the circulation is depressed, the blood moves sluggishly through the system, because it is not purified and vitalized by the pure, invigorating air of heaven. The mind becomes depressed and gloomy, while the whole system is enervated; and fevers and other acute diseases are liable to be generated. (Testimonies for the Church, vol. 1, pp. 702, 703)*

*Air is the free blessing of heaven, calculated to electrify the whole system. (Healthful Living, p. 71)*

---

[10] See Zack Smith, "5 advantages of getting fresh air," published on June 25, 2019, available at https://1ref.us/1t7, accessed 11/27/20.

# CHAPTER 11

# Black Beans[11]

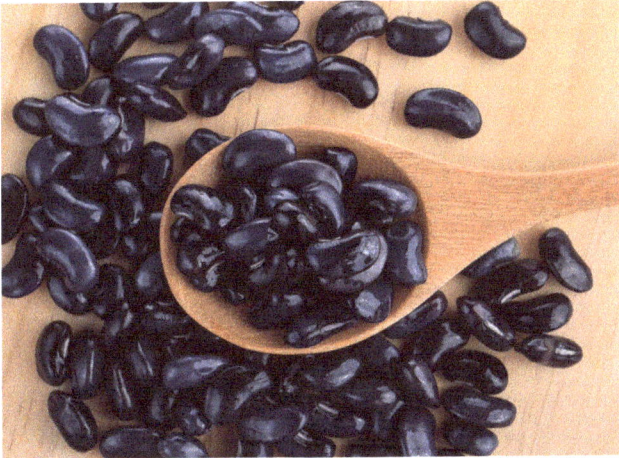

Originating from South America, more than 70% of the calories in black beans are carbs. A large portion is in the form of "resistant starch."

This resistant starch passes through our upper digestive tract without being absorbed, hence it is not converted into simple sugars, and the person's blood sugar levels can avoid an upsurge. Thus, black beans are low on the glycemic index.

Black beans also provide phytonutrients that can be found in deep colored vegetables. Consider black beans in the same category as red cabbage, red onions, or even blueberries.

Black beans have a wholesome 15 grams of fiber and protein per cup and are one of the highest sources of zinc, which improves metabolism. Black beans reduce cholesterol blood levels. The USDA recommends 3 cups per week.

When cooking black beans, do not add salty or acidic seasonings until the beans have been cooked, otherwise they will be tough, increasing cooking time.

---

[11] Joy Stephenson-Laws, "The Benefits of Black Beans Will Blow You Away," available at https://1ref.us/1t8, accessed 12/1/20.

To keep healthy, a sufficient supply of nourishing food is required. With wise planning, that which is most conducive to health can be secured almost everywhere. The various preparations of rice, wheat, corn, oats, beans, peas, and lentils give many choices for a healthy diet. (See *Counsels for the Church*, p. 222.)

# CHAPTER 12

# Blueberries[12]

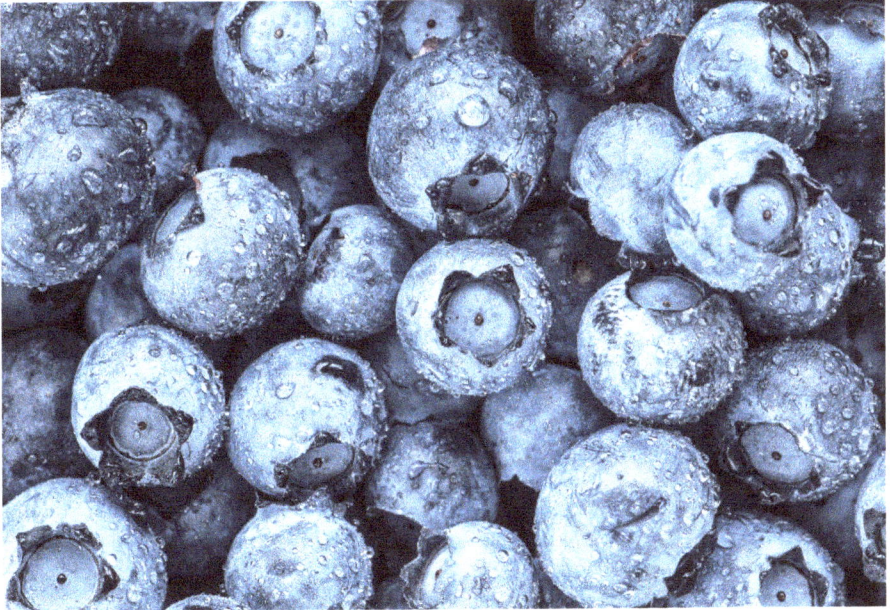

Blueberries rank highest among various foods for antioxidants, which are free-radical-fighting powerhouses. (Free radicals destroy the cells' protection against cancer.) Carrying an abundance of antioxidants known as flavonoids, they can help to reverse age-related memory loss.

Their distinct deep blue and red color is due to a high anthocyanin content. The anthocyanins also neutralize cancer-causing free radicals and can block the growth of tumor cells.

Blueberries and cranberries contain compounds that stop bacteria from sticking to bladder walls and prevent urinary-tract infections (UTIs).

Blueberries have less than 100 calories per cup, but that one cup delivers 14% of the recommended daily intake of fiber and almost 25% of the recommended intake of Vitamin C.

[12] Meenakshi Nagdeve, "20 Evidence-Based Health Benefits Of Blueberries," updated June 30, 2020, available at https://www.organicfacts.net/health-benefits/fruit/health-benefits-of-blueberries.html, accessed 12/4/20.

North America is the leading producer of blueberries, accounting for up to 90% of the world's supply.

> *And this shall be a sign unto thee, Ye shall eat this year such things as grow of themselves, and in the second year that which springeth of the same; and in the third year sow ye, and reap, and plant vineyards, and eat the fruits thereof.* (2 Kings 19:29)

# CHAPTER 13

# Brain Fog[13]

Brain fog is a type of cognitive dysfunction involving memory problems, lack of clarity, poor concentration, and an inability to focus. Some people also describe it as mental fatigue.

Here are six possible causes.

1. Stress. Chronic stress can cause mental fatigue. An exhausted brain has difficulty reasoning and focusing.

2. Lack of sleep. Too little sleep leads to poor concentration and muddled thoughts.

3. Hormonal changes. Changes in the levels of progesterone and estrogen can trigger brain fog. For example, during menopause, a drop in estrogen levels can cause forgetfulness, poor concentration, and cloudy thinking.

4. Diet. A vitamin B12 deficiency can trigger brain fog, as can food allergies or sensitivities. MSG, aspartame, peanuts, and dairy products are common causes. Dehydration can also contribute to reduced mental capacity.

> *Dehydration can also contribute to reduced mental capacity.*

5. Medication.

6. Medical conditions such as anemia, depression, diabetes, migraines, and Alzheimer's disease or autoimmune diseases, such as lupus, arthritis, multiple sclerosis, and hypothyroidism, can also cause brain fog.

To help reduce brain fog:

- Get eight to nine hours of sleep per night.

---

[13] Michael J. Breus, "The Real Reason You Have Brain Fog (And How To Get Rid Of It)," Oct. 10, 2020, available at https://1ref.us/1ta, accessed 12/6/20.

- Manage stress by knowing your limitations.
- Avoid alcohol and caffeine and drink eight glasses of water per day.
- Exercise.
- Strengthen brain power (volunteer or solve brain puzzles).
- Find enjoyable activities.
- Increase intake of protein, fruits, vegetables, and plant-based fats.
- Take supplements. For example, iron supplements can help an anemic person increase the production of red blood cells, which carry more oxygen to the brain and reduce brain fog.

*The mind controls the whole man. All our actions, good or bad, have their source in the mind. It is the mind that worships God, and allies us to heavenly beings. ... All the physical organs are the servants of the mind, and the nerves are the messengers that transmit its orders to every part of the body, guiding the motions of the living machinery....* (*Special Testimonies on Education*, p. 33)

*God desires us, by strict temperance, to keep the mind clear and keen that we may be able to distinguish between the sacred and the common. We should strive to understand the wonderful science of the matchless compassion and benevolence of God.* (*Mind, Character, and Personality*, vol. 2, p. 390)

# CHAPTER **14**

# Children Playing Outside[14]

Today's children may be the first generation at risk for a shorter lifespan than their parents. A sedentary indoor lifestyle has contributed to numerous health problems. Chronic conditions such as childhood obesity, asthma, and ADD have increased over the past few decades. These conditions contribute to pulmonary, cardiovascular, and mental health problems in adulthood.

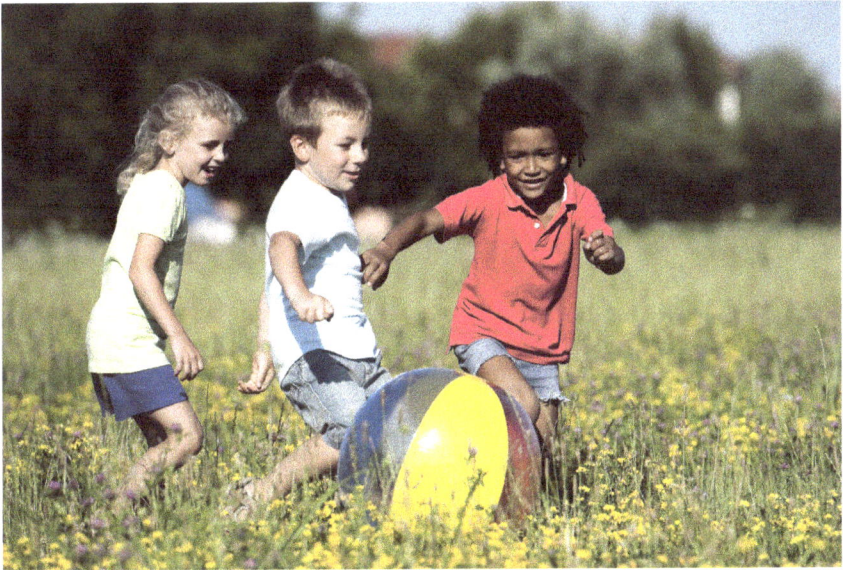

Vitamin D deficiency is responsible for many health problems, but simply going outside for 10–15 minutes of sunlight exposure twice a week can produce the amount of vitamin D our bodies require. Vitamin D can help reduce the severity of asthma in some cases. About 70% (~58.4 million) of US children and adolescents have insufficient levels of vitamin D.

Outdoor activity in nature has been replaced by television, video games, computer usage, and demanding school and extracurricular activities

---

[14] Darryl Edwards, "THE 5 AMAZING BENEFITS OF OUTDOOR EXERCISE [INFOGRAPHIC]," published Jan. 27, 2017, https://1ref.us/1tb, accessed 12/6/20.

schedules. By losing contact with the natural environment, today's youth are missing opportunities for physical activity, releasing stress, restoring focus, and healthy development.

Unstructured outdoor playtime is important for children's overall well-being. Many children's health organizations suggest at least an hour of physical activity a day, which can include unstructured play and walking. They discourage excessive passive entertainment such as TV, Internet, and video games.

The Bible encourages us to care for our children:

*"See that you do not despise one of these little ones. For I tell you that in heaven their angels always see the face of my Father who is in heaven."* (Matthew 18:10, ESV)

# Chapter 15

# Coconut Oil[15]

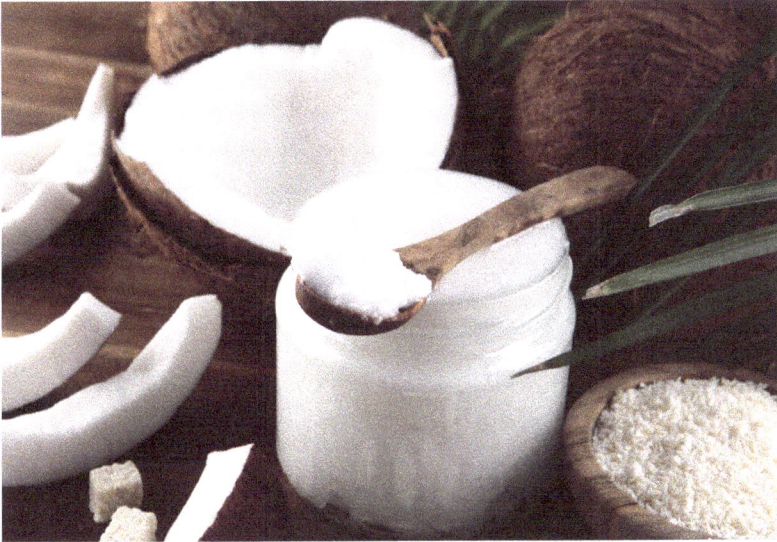

Coconut oil has recently risen to super food status. Various health claims have been made for products such as coconut milk, virgin coconut oil, and coconut cream. In particular, it has been lauded as a cure for Alzheimer's disease, arthritis, diabetes, and both viral and bacterial infections, as well as a booster to the immune system, a useful aid in weight management by burning fat and in preventing heart disease. While many more health claims have been made for coconut oil, insufficient scientific evidence exists to support them all.

Coconut water is the clear liquid inside immature coconuts. It contains sugars and fiber with a small quantity of vitamins and minerals and potassium, in particular. Coconut milk is made by blending water with shredded coconut.

Often, the coconut's milk is 70% water, with over 50% of its calories coming from saturated fat. Coconut cream is a high fat version of coconut

_____
[15] Ashley May, "Think coconut oil is good for your health? Here's what the experts are saying," published Jan. 22, 2020, available at https://1ref.us/1tc, accessed 12/6/20.

milk. Virgin coconut oil (VCO) can be extracted from fresh coconut flesh by grating it and then putting it through a manual press to extract the oil.

- Coconut oil has been called the healthiest oil, perfect for healthy cooking.

- Coconut oil contains 12 grams of saturated fat per tablespoon (85–90% of its calories).

- Coconut oil contains about the same caloric value as all other vegetable oils.

- The saturated fat in coconut can increase LDL and total cholesterol levels. Coconut oil can raise the risk of cardiovascular ailments.

Indigenous populations who include coconut in their traditional cuisine consume a lot of vegetables, fruits, and fish, and they are more active than westerners. They tend to use the high-fiber coconut flesh or coconut milk, but they seldom use coconut oil. Historically these populations have had lower rates of heart disease.

Remember that moderation in the use of even good food is essential. The Bible says, "*Let your moderation be known unto all men. The Lord is at hand*" (Philippians 4:5).

# CHAPTER 16

# Eat Healthy When Traveling[16]

Many of us have traveled, are traveling, or will be traveling. When we are on the road, it is challenging to eat healthy foods. We usually get something quick and easy.

Between pit stops at mini-marts and fast food at an airport, traveling can unravel even the best diet plans. However, with a little preparation and resolve, you can arrive at your destination feeling good about what you consumed along the way. You can do this by taking time to pack some snacks in your carry-on before you leave. Here are some items to include:

- Whole or dried fruit
- Nuts, portioned into snack-size bags
- Whole-grain pretzels or crackers
- Homemade trail mix in one-cup serving containers
- High-fiber granola bars
- Peanut butter crackers

If you can't pack healthy snacks, you can find much of the above at any store. Buying perishables, such as a packaged salad, is another smart way to maintain nutritional standards.

Road trip snacks. One tip for road trips is to pack a cooler with healthy nibbles before you leave. Fill it with fruits, prechopped veggies and hummus dip, and whole-grain sandwiches.

Of course, you'll have pit stops to gas up and use the restroom. If you walk into a convenience store, avoid candy and soda. Instead, reach for whole-grain crackers and bottled water. At a drive-through, you can now enjoy vegetarian burgers, kid-sized upon request, and water instead of soda.

Hotel hacks for healthy eating. When overnighting in a hotel, request a room with a minifridge, then walk to the local grocery store for some

---

[16] Mayo Clinic Staff, "Fast food: Tips for choosing healthier options," May 21, 2021, available at https://1ref.us/1td, accessed 8/3/21.

staples. Does your room have a coffee maker? You can use its hot water to make instant oatmeal in the morning.

> *One tip for road trips is to pack a cooler with healthy nibbles before you leave.*

The motel might even offer a free continental breakfast. Take advantage of this perk, choosing a whole-grain cereal (like oatmeal) with fruit.

Make good restaurant choices. Restaurant meals are almost always higher in calories, fat, and salt than what we prepare at home. Just keep these healthy eating tips in mind:

- Review the menu before sitting down. If it's too greasy, try another restaurant.
- Choose items that are grilled, steamed, baked, or broiled.
- Avoid high-calorie pasta, burritos, or stews.
- Ordering a salad? Ask for a vinaigrette-based dressing on the side.
- At a buffet-style restaurant, aim to fill half of your plate with fruits and vegetables and whole-grain foods.

*The LORD will keep you from all evil; he will keep your life. The LORD will keep your going out and your coming in from this time forth and forevermore.* (Psalm 121:7, 8, ESV)

# CHAPTER 17

# Fasting[17]

Fasting is the process of eliminating either food, drink, or both for a time. An absolute fast is the abstinence from all food and liquids for a period of 24 hours to several days. A person is assumed to be fasting after 8–12 hours without food.

There may be health complications with long-term fasting, such as electrolyte imbalances, thinning hair, cardiac arrhythmia, and renal failure. However, benefits of fasting include reduced risk of cancer, cardiovascular diseases, diabetes, insulin resistance, and autoimmune disorders. Fasting can also slow aging and increase one's lifespan.

Fasting is mentioned numerous times in the Bible:

*Then your light will break forth like the dawn, and your healing will quickly appear; then your righteousness will go before you, and the glory of the LORD will be your rear guard. Then you will call, and the LORD will answer; you will cry for help, and he will say: Here am I.... then your light will rise in the darkness, and your night will become like the noonday.* (Isaiah 58:8–10, NIV)

[17] Nathan Hewitt, "10 Benefits of Fasting That Will Surprise You," available at https://1ref.us/1te, accessed 12/6/20.

# CHAPTER 18

# Fill Your Mouth with Laughter[18]

*He will yet fill your mouth with laughing, and your lips with rejoicing.*
(Job 8:21, NKJV)

Laughter may indeed be the best medicine. In his book, *Anatomy of an Illness*, Norman Cousins recounts how ten minutes of belly laughter gave him two hours of pain-free sleep. Laughter stimulates heart and blood circulation, promotes respiration, produces deep relaxation, and relieves tension.

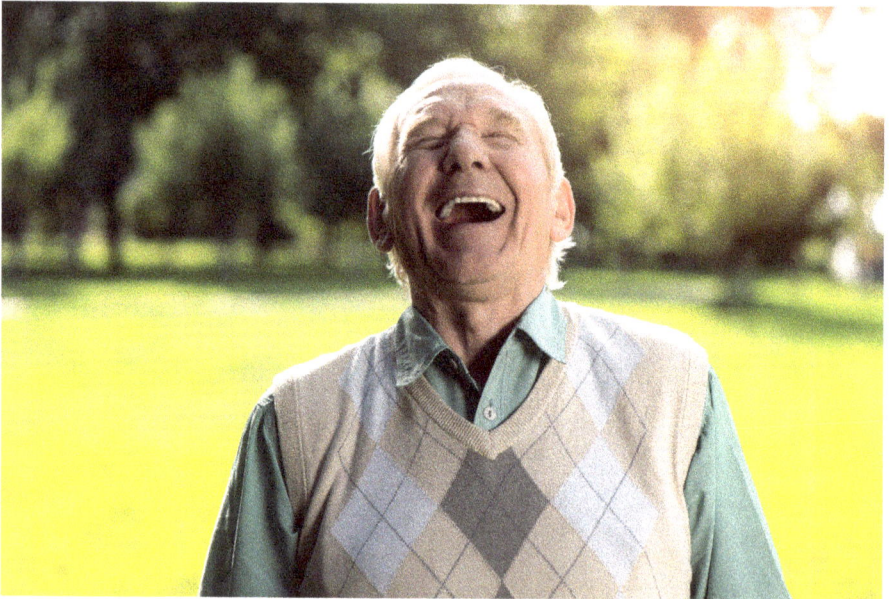

Even putting on a smile can be rewarding. An article in the *Orlando Sentinel* states: "If we just assume facial expressions of happiness, we can increase blood flow to the brain and stimulate release of favorable neurotransmitters." So, a smile we can make us and others around us feel better.

---

[18] Hara Estroff Marano, "Laughter: The Best Medicine," *Psychology Today*, available at https://1ref.us/1tf, accessed 12/6/20.

In addition to laughing and smiling, avoid negative people or "energy vampires" who can drain your energy and enjoyment of life.

God wants us to laugh and enjoy the full range of positive emotions. This is why He promised to "fill your mouth with laughter and your lips with rejoicing"!

So rattle those funny bones today and praise our heavenly Father for the wonderful gift of laughter.

If ten minutes of laughter helped Norman Cousins sleep pain-free for two hours, what could it do for you?

*Norman Cousins recounts how ten minutes of belly laughter gave him two hours of pain-free sleep.*

# CHAPTER 19

# Foods That Fight Cancer[19]

Fill your grocery cart with these powerful and colorful fruits and vegetables, which keep cancer at bay.

Brassicas, like cabbage, cauliflower, brussels sprouts, broccoli, and kale, all help protect against colon cancer. (Broccoli sprouts contain 10 times more cancer-protective substances than mature broccoli.) A higher consumption of green leafy vegetables decreases the risk of breast and skin cancer.

Fruits rich in red pigments, like tomatoes, watermelon, guava, papaya, and pomegranates, provide protection against prostate cancer. Blueberries can suppress colon cancer.

The red, blue, and purple pigments in blackberries, strawberries, raspberries, blueberries, plums, cherries, red grapes, and cranberries also protect against cancer. The deeper the color of the fruit, the stronger the protection.

Carrots and celery contain compounds that have anti-inflammatory, antibiotic, and anti-clotting properties. Studies show these compounds can also slow the growth of colon tumors.

Quercetin is a powerful bioflavonoid found in apples, onions, red grapes, and green leafy vegetables. It is useful for its unique anticancer, antioxidant, and anti-inflammatory activity.

Food does more than fill our tummies; God has provided us with these blessings to keep us healthy.

---

[19] Jamie Eske, "The best cancer-fighting foods," available at https://1ref.us/1tg, accessed 12/6/20.

# CHAPTER 20

# Gallstones vs. Kidney Stones: How Similar Are They?

The purpose of the kidney is to filter blood and then dispose of the wastes by creating urine. The job of the gallbladder is to store bile that helps in the digestion and absorption of fats. Both of these organs can produce a stone.

A kidney stone is a solid mass made up of tiny crystals from minerals like calcium.

Gallstones are pebble-like deposits of cholesterol that form inside the gallbladder. They can be as small as a grain of sand or as large as a golf ball. More than one stone can develop in a kidney or in the gallbladder at the same time.

Women over the age of 40 with diabetes, people who are overweight, or people who have lost weight rapidly are more likely to have gallstones.

Kidney stones occur more in men over 40. A person with one stone has a higher chance of developing another over the next ten years after the first.

With gallstones, a person may experience pain in the upper right abdomen, back pain, nausea, or vomiting.

Conversely, the pain of a kidney stone feels like sharp cramps near the kidneys. Nausea or vomiting and blood in the urine are also symptoms. Small stones often pass on their own. The patient can stay home and drink liquids and take pain medication until the stone passes. If the pain is too severe, the stone can be removed by a medical procedure.

To prevent both types of stones, you should maintain a healthy lifestyle, not skip meals, limit animal protein, and exercise regularly, drinking plenty of water throughout the day.

It's important to get medical attention if you're experiencing symptoms that might be gallstones or kidney stones. To avert these problems, recall the three Hebrew boys who only asked for vegetables, grains, and water during their testing period.[20]

---

[20] AdventHealth, "Gallstones vs Kidney Stones: How Similar Are They?" Sept. 5, 2019, https://1ref.us/1th, accessed 8/3/21.

# CHAPTER 21

# General Facts about Cancer[21]

The symptoms of any type of cancer will depend on where it is, how big it is, and how much it affects the surrounding organs or tissues. If a cancer has spread (metastasized), symptoms may appear in different parts of the body. As a tumor grows, it can create pressure on nearby organs, blood vessels, and nerves. This pressure causes some of the symptoms of cancer. If the cancer is in a critical area, such as certain parts of the brain, even the smallest tumor can cause warning signs. But sometimes it starts in places where it doesn't cause symptoms until it has grown.

Cancer may cause symptoms like fever, extreme fatigue, or weight loss. Cancer consumes much of the body's energy supply and releases substances that change the way the body makes energy from food.

Sometimes it's possible to detect cancer before symptoms appear. The American Cancer Society and other health groups recommend check-ups and certain tests even though there are no symptoms. This helps find certain cancers early before symptoms start.

However, some people ignore symptoms or may be frightened by the thought of having cancer, so they avoid seeking medical advice. But no symptom should be ignored or overlooked, especially if it has lasted a long time or is getting worse.

Treatment works best when cancer is found early—while it's still small and hasn't spread to other parts of the body. Finding it early often means a better chance for survival, especially if the cancer can be removed with surgery.

---

[21] The American Cancer Society medical and editorial content team, "Signs and Symptoms of Cancer," revised Nov. 6, 2020, available at https://1ref.us/1ti, accessed 10/16/20.

# CHAPTER 22

# Good Fats and Oils[22]

First, with fats and oils, remember to let your use of them be sparse.

Fats and oils are high in calories, but they do carry fat-soluble nutrients. Most of our foods have fats as a part of their composition, so we don't need to ingest more to supplement. A little oil, however, can enhance flavors. In the fast-food arena, though, many individuals have health problems due to the high intake of fats.

Some of the most healthful fat is provided by nuts, avocados, legumes, and grains. Eating unprocessed foods yields a balanced fat intake, but a little extra oil or fat is not harmful.

One suggestion is to stop purchasing butter because it is a saturated fat that is tough on blood vessels, and it is not the only spread for bread. Select a margarine with care, avoiding those that contain partially hydrogenated fats, which have been spoiled through their processing. Also, avoid trans fats. Margarines that are healthful are aplenty, but be sure to check the labels.

The secret is to use small amounts. Two tablespoons would represent a full day's requirement, and, because we tend to consume high-fat diets, being vigilant is prudent. It is best to obtain no more than 25 percent of our daily calories from fat sources.

This means minding dairy products. Low-fat varieties are the best.

Use some olive oil or flaxseed oil on salads, even to flavor your cooking.

---

[22] Lawrence Robinson, Jeanne Segal, and Robert Segal, M.A., "Choosing Healthy Fats," last updated October 2020, available at https://1ref.us/1tj, accessed 12/1/20.

# Chapter 23

# Gratitude[23]

According to Dr. Art Calhoun, being grateful can have health benefits, such as low blood pressure and being happy.[24] By beginning a gratitude journal, you can establish the daily practice of paying attention to gratitude-inspiring events and writing them down.

*Choosing to associate with grateful individuals can be a positive influence.*

Visual reminders, such as Post-It notes, can be placed on a refrigerator, mirror, or steering wheel, to jog your memory to list your blessings.

A "gratitude partner" can support and encourage you to discipline yourself to adopt healthier behaviors. Choosing to associate with grateful individuals can be a positive influence. Find someone who is grateful and spend more time with that person.

Other ways to focus on gratitude include making a public commitment to write in a journal and changing your self-talk by using positive affirmations.

Last, but not least, pray! Ask to be shown the numerous blessings the Lord bestows on you every day.

In *The Adventist Home*, Mrs. White acknowledged, "Troubles may invade, but these are the lot of humanity. Let patience, gratitude, and love keep sunshine in the heart though the day may be ever so cloudy" (p. 18).

---

[23] Kori D. Miller, "14 Health Benefits of Practicing Gratitude According to Science," *Positive Psychology.com*, Feb. 27, 2021, available at https://1ref.us/1tk, accessed 12/6/20.
[24] Dr. Art Calhoun (family medicine physician), "Gratitude," September 21, 2013, a health lecture at the Frostburg Seventh-day Adventist Church, West Union, WV.

# CHAPTER 24

# Guavas[25]

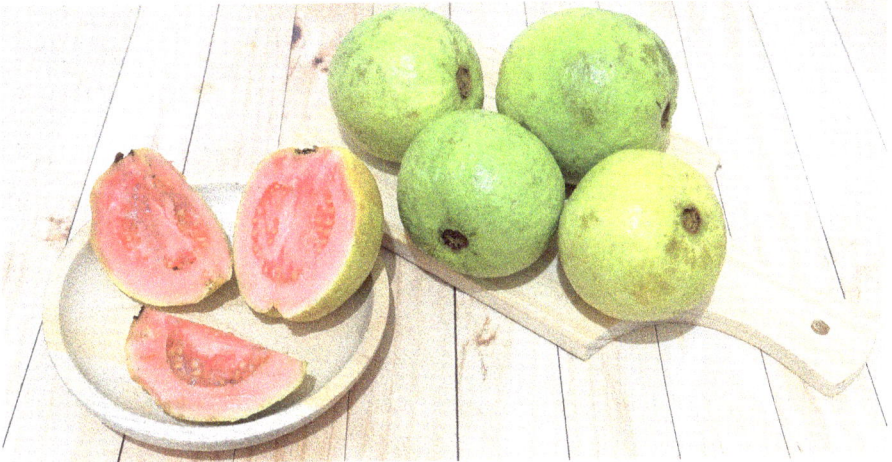

Native to Mexico, Central America, and northern South America, this fruit is round with a green exterior and a pink interior. It tastes like a pear and is full of edible seeds. Guava is usually eaten raw like an apple.

Guava grows in warmer temperatures but is one of the few plants that will fruit while potted indoors. The entire fruit can be used for punch, while the juice is used in sauces, candies, dried snacks, fruit bars, and desserts. The high levels of pectin make it a popular choice for preserves, jams, and jellies.

Guavas are rich in dietary fiber and vitamin C. One guava fruit contains about four times as much vitamin C as an orange. It also contains essential minerals, such as calcium, phosphorus, magnesium, iron, and potassium, and has moderate levels of folic acid. Guava is a good source of copper, and it is important for regulating metabolism, controlling hormone production, and absorbing nutrients.

Vitamin C is known to help prevent cancer, regulate blood pressure, and treat diarrhea. It also aids in weight loss, improves the skin, and

---

[25] Dan Lewis, "15 Fruity Facts About Guavas," *The Fact Site*, last updated Aug. 3, 2021, available at https://1ref.us/1tl, accessed 12/6/20.

mitigates coughs and colds, constipation, dysentery, and scurvy. Guava is a low carb, high fiber food, and it has no cholesterol.

If you see guavas for sale in the market, give them a try.

*And God said, "Let the earth sprout vegetation, plants yielding seed, and fruit trees bearing fruit in which is their seed, each according to its kind, on the earth." And it was so.* (Genesis 1:11, ESV)

# CHAPTER 25

# H$_2$O[26]

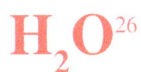

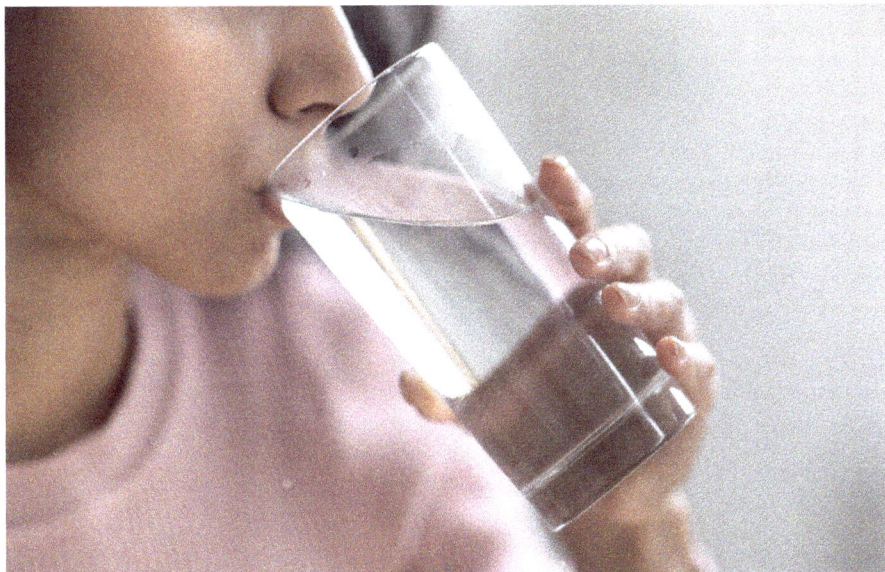

Our bodies are 2/3 water. Thus, it is the main element of human composition. Water—

- Moisturizes the air in the lungs
- Boosts metabolism
- Helps absorb nutrients better
- Regulates body temperature
- Detoxifies
- Protects and moisturizes our joints.

*To quench thirst, pure water is all that nature requires.*

Drinking water helps you lose weight because it flushes out the by-products of fat breakdown. Water is an effective appetite suppressant. Water—

---

[26] Lauren Holway, "How Drinking Enough Water Improves Your Health," updated July 20, 2021, available at https://1ref.us/1tm, accessed 8/3/21.

- Is a natural remedy for headache
- Produces healthier skin
- Improves productivity at work
- Improves the quality of one's exercise
- Helps in digestion and constipation
- Is responsible for less cramps and sprains
- Makes a person less likely to get sick and more likely to feel healthy
- Relieves fatigue
- Supports a pleasant mood
- Reduces the risk of cancer

To quench thirst, pure water is all that nature requires. Never drink tea, coffee, beer, wine, or spirituous liquors.

# CHAPTER 26

# The Healthiest Sugar[27]

Sugar, in particular the bright white, refined type, has always been a nutritional no-no. Although it is a purified form of the sucrose that comes from sugar cane or beets, in its refined form, it spikes blood sugar, increases inflammation, and offers an endless roller coaster of cravings. The artificial substitutes for refined sugar, such as Splenda® and Sweet'N Low®, are toxic, and it is best to avoid them.

Brown sugar, or raw sugar is, white sugar's rustic cousin. It can be less refined, and it contains some of the sugar cane's molasses. Nutritionally, the differences between white and brown sugar are trivial. The molasses that is added back into brown sugar, however, contains calcium, iron, and potassium, yet not enough to make it a significant source of any of these. The molasses imparts a unique flavor and texture, but it doesn't make it more healthful. It is less processed—which means it hasn't been bleached or boiled—which is probably better for the planet.

Besides these, there are other sugars:

- Agave nectar, which comes from several species of agave plant
- Barley malt, which comes from sprouted barley
- Brown rice syrup
- Date sugar
- Maple syrup
- Maple sugar
- Palm sugar
- Honey
- Molasses

Yet, the big question still remains: What kind of sugar should I use?

Our bodies do not need refined sugar, and limiting sugar intake can make a positive impact on overall health. The next time that a recipe calls for sugar, give raw honey, barley malt, brown rice syrup, or blackstrap molasses a try.

---

[27] Vasanti Malik, ScD., "Are certain types of sugars healthier than others?" May 29, 2019, available at https://1ref.us/1tn, accessed 12/12/20.

# CHAPTER 27

# Heart Health[28]

February is the month to recognize the health of our hearts.

The risk factors for heart disease for men and women are high blood pressure, elevated cholesterol levels, smoking, lack of physical activity, obesity, diabetes, family history of heart disease, sex, age, stress and use of alcohol.

The American Heart Association recommends these six lifestyle changes:

1.  Avoid smoking.
2.  Monitor high blood pressure.
3.  Lower your intake of cholesterol and saturated fats.
4.  Increase your physical activity.
5.  Maintain a healthy weight.
6.  Have regular medical exams

Medical professionals suggests these steps to have a healthy heart. Perhaps a seventh item belongs on this list: trust, love, and obey God. The heart of the matter—the truth of the matter—is that the greatest commandment that God our Creator has given us is to "love the Lord your God with all your heart, soul, mind and strength, and to love others as yourself. "

Loving God from the bottom of our heart can transform us. When we accept his love and forgiveness for all our wrongdoings and sins, we can experience His deep love. Genuine peace comes from complete trust in Him. Believe that the Holy Bible is truth and follow God's principles for living to experience the full life that He desires for us all. This includes a healthy spiritual heart and a healthy physical heart.

*"Above all else, guard your heart, for it is the wellspring of* life."
(Proverbs 4:23)

---

[28] "7 Proven Ways To Keep Your Heart Healthy," *News on Heart.org*, https://safebeat.org/cardiac/heart_health/7_ways_to_keep_heart_healthy/, accessed 12/6/20.

# CHAPTER 28

# Honey[29]

Honey has about the same relative sweetness as granulated sugar, but also contains tiny amounts of compounds that function as antioxidants, including vitamin C.

The antioxidants in honey are used for treatment of sore throats, coughs, and allergies. Dark colored honey has higher antioxidant content.

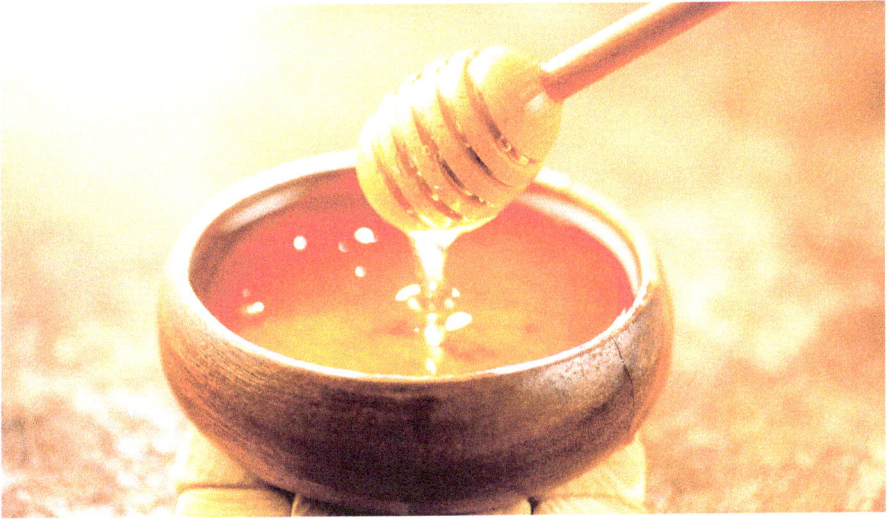

Another function of honey involves the treatment of wounds. This technique involves placing honey on the patient's wounds to prevent infection. When honey "ointment" is applied to ulcerated surfaces it stimulates a profuse flow of lymph, which soaks the entire surface of the wound. This liquid is not only antibacterial but it cleanses the wounds and stimulates and promotes granulation and healing. The treatment reduces inflammation and prevents deep tissue death. It is well tolerated because it alleviates pain and eases tension. Dressing changes are not painful because the lymph fluid prevents the dressing material from sticking to the wound and it can be removed with ease.

---

[29] "Honey Can Help Wound Healing," *Advanced Tissue*, available at https://www.ncbi.nlm.nih.gov/pmc/articles/PMC6027142/, accessed 12/6/20.

## CHAPTER 29

# Laughter Can Improve Short-Term Memory[30]

When we laugh, the stress hormone cortisol decreases and our short-term memory improves.

Have you ever forgotten where you put your keys? Or maybe it was that one word that was at the tip of your tongue? Short-term memory loss can be common, especially when we're stressed.

Loma Linda University Health researchers have found that, when we are tense, our cortisol levels increase. Cortisol is a stress hormone and, when it enters our brain, it can damage neurons involved with learning and memory.

A number of people were divided into two groups. One watched a 20-minute video that made them laugh. The other just sat in the waiting room. The humor group had decreased cortisol levels as compared to the non-humor group.

Lower your stress levels by laughing more. Socialize with friends. Plan to do something enjoyable after work. When we laugh, the stress hormone cortisol decreases and our short-term memory will improve.

*A joyful heart is good medicine, but a crushed spirit dries up the bones.* (Proverbs 17:22, ESV)

---

[30] Janelle Ringer, "Laughter: A fool-proof prescription," April 1, 2019, available at https://1ref.us/1to, accessed 12/6/20.

# CHAPTER 30

# Lentils[31]

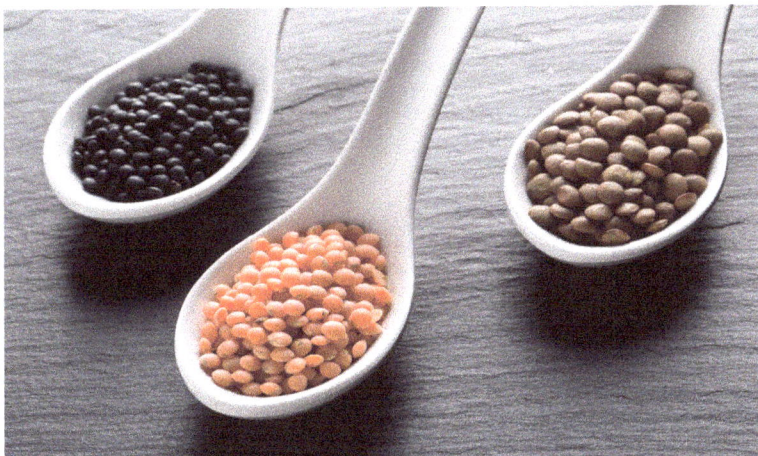

Lentils have been part of the human diet for a long time, and they are some of the most nutritious and, at the same time, most economical foods in the world.

These legumes are grown like peas in a pod, and they come in a wide array of colors including brown, pink, green, and orange.

They are commonplace in Eastern Europe, in India, and in parts of Asia.

Whatever color you choose, lentils are low in fat, low in calories, and free from cholesterol. They are often combined with rice, which has a similar cooking time.

With about 30% of their calories from protein, lentils have the third-highest level of protein, by weight, of any legume or nut after soybeans and hemp.

Lentils also contain dietary fiber, folate, vitamin B1, and minerals.

They are low in fat and high in fiber, thereby getting rid of cholesterol and reducing blood cholesterol levels to avoid accumulation and buildup of the fat that can lead to heart disease, high blood pressure, and stroke.

---

[31]The Nutrition Source, "Lentils," available at https://1ref.us/1tp, accessed 12/11/20.

Lentils can also slow down the liver's manufacture of cholesterol.

**Improvement for Diabetes.** Doctors often advise those who suffer from diabetes to include lentils in their diet. This is because the large amount of soluble fiber in lentils helps trap carbohydrates, which can slow digestion and absorption and help reduce the risks of spikes in the blood sugar level.

**Boosts Digestion.** With the high levels of fiber in lentils, they also make it easier for the body to get rid of toxins.

CHAPTER **31**

# Mental Health[32]

It's astonishing that *one in five adults and children in the United States struggle with depression, schizophrenia, anxiety disorders, and other incapacities.*

The cause of mental illness is not yet fully understood. Some factors may include a biochemical imbalance, heredity, stress, recreational drug use, or abuse. Mental illness is often temporary, and most people who have it are functioning individuals who are rational as much of the time as they are symptomatic or psychotic.

The types of mental illness are: (1) schizophrenia; (2) dementia or Alzheimer's; (3) mood disorders—depression, bipolar and suicide; (4) anxiety disorders—panic attack, phobias, obsessive-compulsion and post-traumatic stress; (5) personality disorders—antisocial, paranoid and schizoid, narcissistic, histrionic, dependent, and avoidant; (6) eating disorders; (7) autism; and (8) attention deficit disorder or hyperactivity.

So, what can we do about those who have such an illness? We can convey an accepting and genuine manner, and w3e should avoid being judgmental. We should provide an understanding response to the person's concern as a resource for information and referrals, and we should focus on the person's strengths, reminding them that God cares for them.

Deuteronomy 31:8 declares:

*The LORD himself goes before you and will be with you; he will never leave you nor forsake you. Do not be afraid; do not be discouraged.* (NIV)

---

[32] Pathways To Promise Manual, handouts; and National Institute of Mental Health, "PASTORAL CARE FOR PEOPLE WITH MENTAL ILLNESS," https://1ref.us/1tq, accessed 3/15/19.

# CHAPTER 32

# Milk[33]

The news this week announced that the price of milk and other dairy products will increase to as much as $9 a gallon. Sounds like a great time to review some dairy-free milk alternatives!

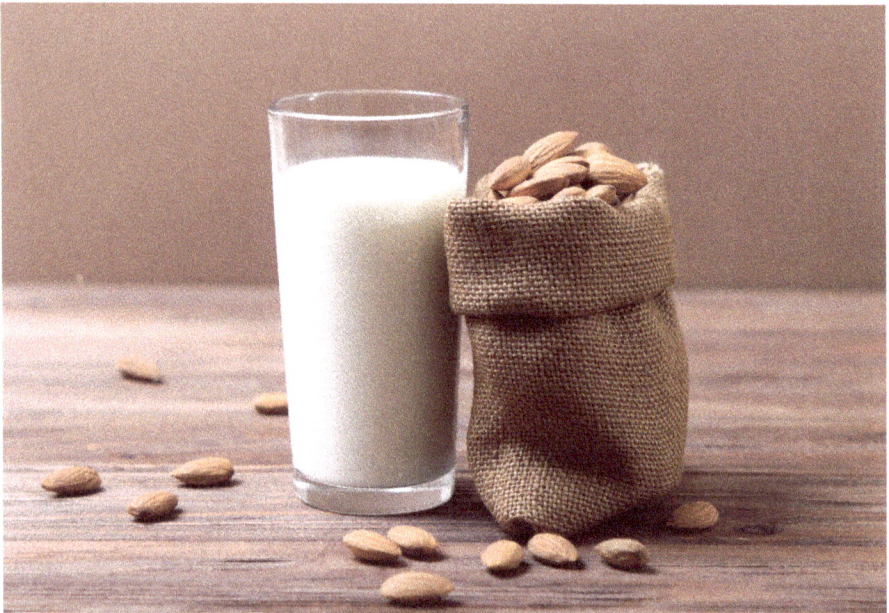

**Rice milk** is not as thick as dairy milk, and it has a somewhat translucent consistency. Because it is sweet, rice milk works well in dessert recipes, but it is not suited for savory or salty dishes, such as mashed potatoes. Compared to soy and almond milk, rice milk has a lower percentage of protein.

 **Hemp milk** is less common, but you can find it in aseptic (non-refrigerated) packs, sometimes near the cereal aisle with other breakfast foods.

 **Milk made from almonds or other nuts**, such as cashew milk, has a creamy consistency similar to soy milk, and it has a nutty taste that is

[33] EcoWatch, "6 Alternatives To Milk: Which Is The Healthiest?" May 2, 2016, available at https://1ref.us/1tr, accessed 12/11/20.

perfect for making vegan fruit smoothies or other drinks and desserts. These nut milks don't taste much like dairy milk, so they are best used in non-savory dishes.

Substitute oat milk, rice milk, or almond milk for the milk ingredient in your recipes. Look for brands that keep the sugar content to twelve grams or less and the sodium content to no more than 100 milligrams per serving. Also, look for the non-genetically modified stamp on the package and for milk without carrageenan. You won't even be able to tell the difference in most recipes.

And, if you have the resources, buy organic almonds, cashews, or oats in bulk, grind them in a blender with water and a pinch of salt and vanilla, and enjoy the healthiest alternative to dairy.

If a recipe calls for buttermilk, add one tablespoon of white vinegar or lemon juice to a cup of soymilk, to replace the buttermilk, and mix well.

As a butter substitute, a non-dairy vegan margarine, such as Earth Balance, will do fine. For cheese, try nutritional yeasts and tofu alternatives.

# CHAPTER 33

# Mustard Greens[34]

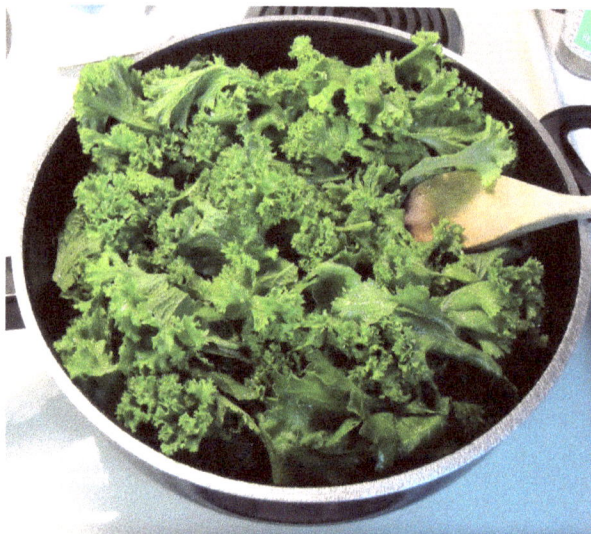

Eating healthy is something to strive for. One way to do this is by becoming familiar with mustard greens. They are just as healthy as the ever-popular kale and can boast of their high levels of antioxidants and their ability to lower cholesterol. With a pungent bite and a peppery flavor, they give your daily dose of greens a nice kick and can add a wonderful dimension to many dishes. They're also wholesome and easy to grow in a garden.

Sauté mustard greens for an easy side dish. Swap them for kale in any of your kale-centric dishes.

Mustard greens are the leaves of the mustard plant (*Brassica juncea*). These often appear in Southern cooking as well as Indian, Chinese, Japanese, and African cuisines.

When choosing mustard greens, know that the smaller, more tender leaves of spring will generally be milder in flavor than the mature leaves of summer and fall. We like mustard greens just lightly wilted, blanched, or sautéed to retain the bright color and texture, but they can also be boiled

---

[34] Malia Frey, "Mustard Greens Nutrition Facts and Health Benefits," available at https://1ref.us/1ts, accessed 12/11/20.

or braised longer to soften the flavor. Ingredients that help balance the taste include salt, soy sauce, toasted nuts, olive oil, or sesame oil.

1. Mustard greens, like spinach, are the storehouse of many **phytonutrients** that have health-promoting and disease-preventing properties.
2. Mustard greens are low in calories and fats. However, their dark-green leaves contain a good amount of **fiber** that helps to control cholesterol levels by interfering with its absorption in the gut.
3. These greens are considered to be one of the highest among leafy vegetables for **vitamin K** and **folic acid.**

Mustard greens have proven benefits against prostatic, breast, colon, and ovarian cancers by virtue of their cancer-cell growth inhibition and cytotoxic effects on cancer cells.

Systematic consumption of mustard greens in the diet is known to prevent arthritis, osteoporosis, and iron deficiency anemia, and it is believed to protect against cardiovascular diseases, asthma, and colon and prostatic cancers.

# CHAPTER 34

# Okra

Also known as "lady's fingers," okra is a flowering plant.

1. Okra belongs to the same family as hibiscus and cotton. The term "okra" refers to the edible seedpods of the plant.
2. Okra contains potassium, vitamin B, vitamin C, folic acid, and calcium. It's low in calories and has a high dietary fiber content.
3. Popular forms for medicinal purposes include okra water, okra peels, and powdered seeds.
4. Roasted okra seeds have been suggested for the management of blood sugar in cases of type 1, type 2, and gestational diabetes.[35]
5. Okra is also a diuretic. It helps the body detoxify and sheds excess water weight. A great aid for de-bloating!

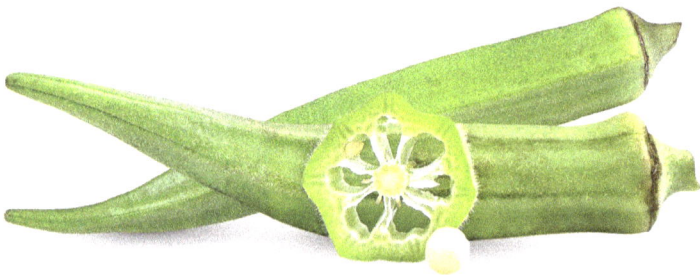

Choose okra that is firm and avoid shriveled or soft pods. Once the pods start turning dark on the ends, they will spoil. Fresh okra can last three to four days.

---

[35] Kathryn Watson and George Krucik, MD, MBA, "Benefits of Okra for Diabetes," updated May 11, 2019, available at https://1ref.us/1tt, accessed 3/8/19.

1. Dried okra can be used to make or thicken a sauce or as an egg white substitute.
2. Okra seeds can also be roasted and ground to make a non-caffeinated coffee substitute.[36]

Sauté okra with tomatoes and onions, or roast it in the oven. It can be flavored with olive oil, salt and pepper, or smothered with spices. Coat it in cornmeal, use an air fryer or your oven on high to fry it. Many cultures simmer it in stews and soups.

One hack that my mom taught me is to squeeze lemon juice in the pan while cooking to break up the slime.

---

[36] Natalie Olsen, "Benefits and uses of okra," *Medical News Today*, Nov. 6, 2019, available at https://1ref.us/1tu, accessed 3/8/19.

# CHAPTER 35

# Pumpkin[37]

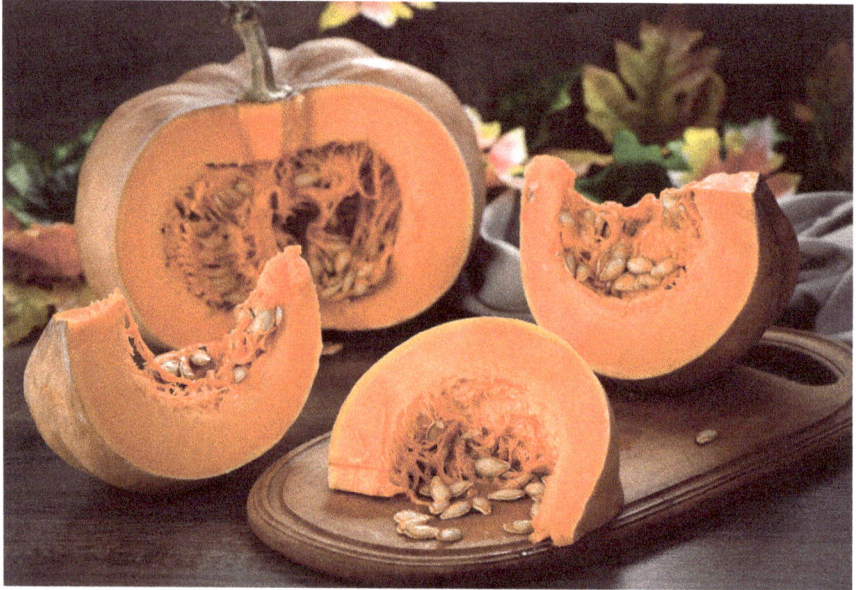

Pumpkin is one of the most nutritious fruits. Loaded with antioxidants and disease-fighting vitamins, these squash-family gourds are a bona fide superfood.

The pumpkin's bright orange color is due to beta-carotene, a provitamin that is converted to vitamin A in the body.

Known for its immune-boosting powers, beta-carotene is essential for eye health and has also been linked to preventing coronary heart disease.

If pumpkins are not in season, one cup of canned pumpkin has seven grams of fiber and three grams of protein—even more than fresh pumpkin—and it contains only 80 calories and one gram of fat.

In addition, canned pumpkin is packed with vitamins and provides over 50 percent of the daily value of vitamin K, which may reduce the risk for some types of cancer.

---

[37] Jaclyn London, "What Are the Health Benefits of Pumpkin? Here's What You Need to Know," *Good Housekeeping*, Sept. 11, 2019, available at https://1ref.us/1tv, accessed 12/5/20.

Canned pumpkin can be added to almost anything. For a hot breakfast filled with fiber, try adding canned pumpkin to oatmeal.

A handy tip: if a recipe calls for canned pumpkin, you can use fresh pumpkin in its place.

Nonetheless, the real treasure is in the seeds. One ounce of pumpkin seeds (about 140 seeds) is packed with protein, magnesium, potassium, and zinc. Studies suggest that pumpkin seeds (also known as "pepitas") provide numerous health benefits—such as blocking the enlargement of the prostate gland, lowering the risk of bladder stones, and preventing depression.

Pumpkin seeds also contain high levels of phytosterols, which research suggests can reduce cholesterol and even help prevent some types of cancers. So, get scooping!

# CHAPTER 36

# Ramps and Wild Onions[38]

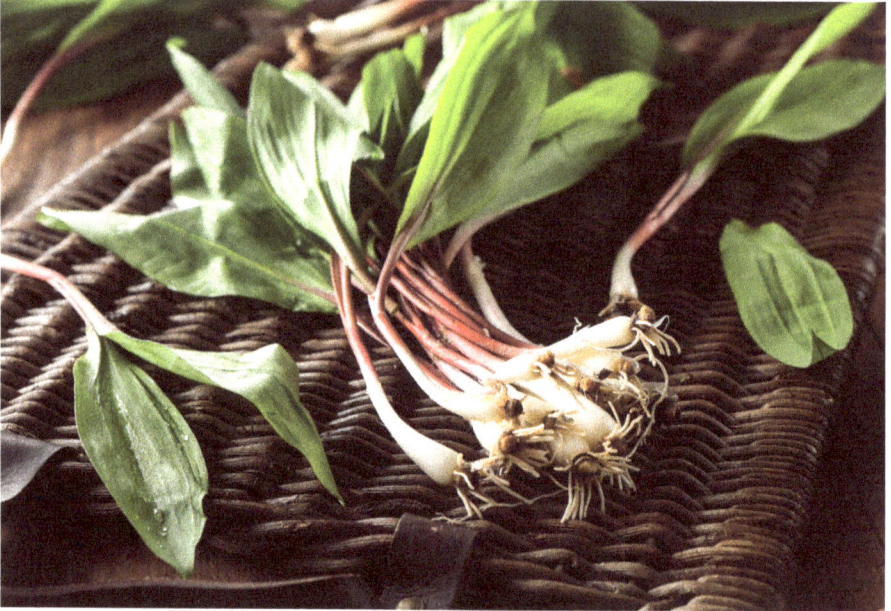

Ramps and wild onions are some of the first vegetables to emerge from the defrosting soil in the spring. Ramps, spring onions, ramsons, wild leeks, wood leeks, and wild garlic thrive in North America, Canada, and the Eastern United States, and they are widespread in Appalachia and in many back yards.

Ramps often grow below the shade of deciduous trees in rich soil. They have light green leaves, often with deep purple lower stems. Both the white lower leaf stalks and the broad green leaves are edible.

Ramps have a garlic-like aroma and a pronounced onion flavor.

In Canada, ramps are delicacies, and selling ramps there commercially can be punishable by fine.

Ramps have similar nutritional content to their cultivated counter parts—leeks. They are high in vitamin A (a one-cup serving satisfying

[38] Julie Daniluk, "Ramp up your heart health with wild leeks," Chatelaine, available at https://1ref.us/1tw, accessed 12/6/20.

30 percent of the recommended daily value) and vitamin E, which are essential to the formation of healthy teeth, bones, skin, and a good working immune system, among other benefits.

Wild onions provide a wealth of minerals such as manganese, iron, and chromium, which are important in metabolizing fats, carbohydrates, and insulin.

Ramps can improve the immune system, lower bad cholesterol levels, and fight cancer.

Onions contain a variety of anti-inflammatory compounds that may improve symptoms of asthma.

The Chippewa Indians decocted the root to induce vomiting, while the Cherokee consumed ramps to remedy colds and made a juice from the plant to treat an earache.

Ramps are most commonly fried with potatoes, can be sprinkled on a salad, or can add flavor to soups and savory dishes.

**Wild Leek and Cashew Pesto**

Ingredients:

- 1 bunch or about 6–8 wild leeks
- 1/2 cup of fresh basil leaves
- 1/2 cup of fresh dill
- 2 garlic cloves
- 1 cup of cashews, soaked overnight or for 4 hours or more
- 1 tbsp of dried oregano
- 1/4 cup of nutritional yeast
- 1/2 cup of filtered water
- Juice of 2 lemons
- 1/4 cup of extra virgin olive oil
- 1 tbsp of coarse sea salt

Directions: In a food processor or high-speed blender, combine all ingredients until the pesto is smooth and creamy. Use as a pasta sauce with your favorite pasta or as a creamy salad dressing.

CHAPTER **37**

# The Science of Junk Food[39]

Salt, fat, and sugar are not consumed by chance; they are consumed by design, though perhaps not by our design sometimes.

Processed foods in the grocery stores have been *engineered* to fool the body's natural hunger and stop the "fullness feeling signal."

According to a recent *New York Times* article, these foods have been formulated and tested to maximize enjoyment and minimize fullness or the desire to stop eating (called the "bliss point").

Be alert for "low-fat" processed food in particular. The fat is often replaced with sugar to add flavor, but sugars and other high-carb grains are more challenging than fat consumption.

Higher and more harmful calorie-dense food infused with addictive flavors and sensations cause you to crave more.

In God's design, however, "a bondservant of Christ should eat and drink all to the glory of God—using only 'that which is good'" (Isaiah 55:2).[40]

---

[39] Michael Moss, "The Extraordinary Science Of Addictive Junk Food," available at https://1ref.us/1tx, accessed 12/12/20.
[40] Richard Anthony, "Biblical Health Principles," available at https://1ref.us/1ty, accessed 8/4/21.

# CHAPTER 38

# Simple and Effective Ways to Avoid Getting Sick[41]

Nutrition makes all the difference to a weakened immune system. To prevent illness, drink plenty of fluids—dehydrated mucous surfaces are a breeding ground for viruses. Sugar depresses immune functions. Increased levels of sugar reduce vitamin C levels. Even fruit juice, like orange juice, can depress immune function. Studies show that sugar of all kinds impairs the ability of white blood cells to kill bacteria and that it weakens the immune system and competes with vitamin C.

In addition to avoiding sugar, it is vital to keep away from dairy and other mucous forming foods like gluten, in particular, if you are susceptible to illnesses such as colds and sinusitis. These foods create a mucous surface and allow bacteria and viruses to thrive.

*By adding seasonal foods to your plate, you gain essential vitamins and minerals, including antioxidants that defend your body from disease.*

Besides keeping nutrition in mind to stay well, also pay attention to other bodily needs, such as rest. Go to bed early and stay there if you are not feeling well. During deep sleep, strong immune-enhancing compounds are released, and many functions are boosted.

In regard to diet, choose autumn harvest foods, including carrots, sweet potatoes, onions, and garlic. Also emphasize spices and seasonings including ginger, peppercorns, and mustard seeds.

Consider it a principle that foods that take longer to grow are more warming than foods that grow fast. Fruits and vegetables eaten in season have been found to contain more nutrients. Produce bought out of season

---

[41] National Institutes of Health, "How dietary factors influence disease risk," March 14, 2017, available at https://1ref.us/1tz, accessed 11/27/20.

is likely to have been grown in artificial conditions or picked too soon and transported long distances.

By adding seasonal foods to your plate, you gain essential vitamins and minerals, including antioxidants that defend your body from disease.

# CHAPTER **39**

# Sleep Deprivation[42]

Sleep deprivation means that you are not getting enough sleep.

Most adults need seven to eight hours of sleep each night. Less sleep than that can lead to assorted health problems. These can include forgetfulness, being less able to fight off infections, and even mood swings and depression.

Sleep deprivation can occur for a number of reasons:

- A sleep disorder, such as insomnia, sleep apnea, or narcolepsy.
- Persons older than 65 have trouble sleeping because of aging, medicine they're taking, or medical problems they're experiencing.
- Illness–sleep deprivation is common with depression, schizophrenia, chronic pain syndrome, cancer, stroke, and Alzheimer's disease.
- Other factors include stress, a new baby, or a change in schedule.

Initial sleep deprivation symptoms may include:

- Drowsiness
- The inability to concentrate
- Impaired memory
- Reduced physical strength
- A diminished ability to fight off infections

Sleep deprivation complications over time may include:

- Increased risk for depression and mental illness
- Increased risk for stroke and asthma attack
- Increased risk for life-threatening difficulties, such as car accidents, and untreated sleep disorders like insomnia, sleep apnea, and narcolepsy
- Hallucinations
- Severe mood swings

---

[42] Kathleen Davis and Raj Dasgupta, MD, "What to know about sleep deprivation," July 23, 2020, available at https://1ref.us/1u0, accessed 12/12/20.

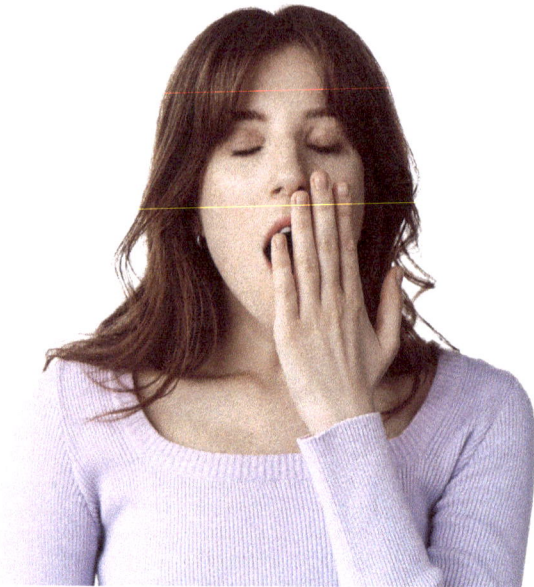

One of the telltale signs of sleep deprivation is feeling lethargic during the day. Also, if you often fall asleep within five minutes of lying down, then you might be experiencing sleep deprivation.

Can sleep deprivation be prevented?

If it is mild, these simple strategies may help you to get a better night's sleep:

- Exercise 20 to 30 minutes each day or more, and at least five to six hours before going to bed. You will be more likely to fall asleep later in the day.

- Avoid substances that contain caffeine, nicotine, and alcohol—all of which can disrupt sleep patterns. Quitting smoking is always a good idea.

In *Manuscript Releases*, volume 9, page 47, Ellen White wrote: "Wake up in the mornings. Set your hour to rise early, and bring yourself to it, then retire at an early hour, and you will see that you will overcome many painful disorders which distress the mind, cause gloomy feelings, discouragement, and unhappy friction, and disqualify you for doing anything without great taxation."

*His disciples replied, "Lord, if he sleeps, he will get better."* (John 11:12, NIV)

CHAPTER **40**

# Social Longevity[43]

Nearly 7,000 individuals living in Alameda County, California, were observed for several years to look at seven lifestyle factors that influenced longevity.

One was how their social relationships affected their mortality.

To the surprise of many skeptics, the research suggested that trusting God and attending church on a regular basis increased lifespan. Having genuine friends, being a member of a group, and even being married have real benefits.

Most individuals recognize that these elements enhance the moral and social quality of life, but they also affect physical health and endurance. Increasing research testifies to the value of belief in God for one's social and emotional well-being.

When the Alameda County study was analyzed for these social and spiritual factors, they found that 30- to 49-years-olds with strong religious faith reported higher levels of happiness. They also appeared to handle traumatic events with less mental and social difficulties, proving how that faith in God enhances a person's health. On the value of corporate gatherings, Ellen G. White wrote:

*When the Alameda County study was analyzed for these social and spiritual factors, they found that 30- to 49-years-olds with strong religious faith reported higher levels of happiness.*

> *We sustain a loss when we neglect the privilege of associating to strengthen and encourage one another in the service of God. The truths of His Word lose their vividness and importance in our minds. Our hearts cease to be enlightened and aroused by their sanctifying*

[43] Jamie Ducharme, "You Asked: Do Religious People Live Longer?" Feb. 15, 2018, available at https://1ref.us/1u1, accessed 12/6/20.

*influence, and we decline in spirituality. In our association as Christians we lose much by lack of sympathy. He who shuts himself up is not filling the position that God designed he should. The proper cultivation of the social elements in our nature brings us into sympathy with others, and is a means of development and strength to us in the service of God. (Steps to Christ,* p. 101)

# CHAPTER 41

# Soluble Fiber[44]

Fiber, which is classified as either insoluble or soluble, is essential to our diet. Soluble fiber, such as oats, barley, legumes, and many fruits, refers to components that dissolve in water to form a gel. This type of fiber decreases the levels of total and LDL cholesterol. Maintaining low cholesterol levels is one way to lower the risk of developing heart disease.

On the other hand, insoluble fiber doesn't dissolve in water. It too is crucial in a healthy diet. It processes through the digestive system slowly enough for nutrients to be absorbed in the intestines but fast enough to prevent constipation. Insoluble and soluble fiber can be obtained in various foods found in a balanced diet. Thus, you should eat a wide variety of natural foods to benefit from both.

Women need about 25 grams of fiber per day, and men need about 38. Twenty-five grams can be gotten in five apples or 80 baby carrots or five and a half large oranges or three and a half cups of shredded coconut or seven cups of blueberries or two cups of peanuts.

**Beans and Seeds.** Many beans contain plenty of soluble fiber. Examples include lima beans, kidney beans, and soybeans. Peas qualify as well, as do cowpeas and lentils. Several seeds have high soluble fiber content too, such as sunflower seeds, flax seeds, and sesame seeds.

**Fruits and Vegetables.** Many fruits and vegetables have a high soluble fiber content such as artichokes, eggplants, broccoli, celery, and carrots, as well as oranges, apples, kiwis, blueberries, tomatoes, strawberries, and bananas.

**Grains and Nuts.** Several grains, including barley, oats, and bran, offer an abundant source of soluble fiber. Nuts, including Brazil nuts and almonds, also have soluble fiber. Fiber works best when absorbed with water.

---

[44] Mayo Clinic Staff, "Dietary fiber: Essential for a healthy diet," Jan. 6, 2021, available at https://1ref.us/1u2, accessed 2/14/19.

# CHAPTER 42

# Summer Fruits and Vegetables[45]

Summer fruits and vegetables are around for a short time, so let's make the most of them. Think simple: they can be lightly cooked, with simple dressings, or eaten raw.

## FRUITS

Summer fruits yield over the course of the summer months. Some of these, like strawberries, diminish from mid-July, while others, don't arrive until later.

- **Apricots.** Eat them fresh, in halves, stuffed and baked, or cook and puree them to use them in ice cream, a mousse, or a soufflé.

- **Blackberries.** Pick them from hedgerows at the end of summer and rinse them thoroughly before use. They are perfect stewed with apples, alone, or in crumbles and pies.

- **Blackcurrants.** The intense flavor of this small fruit is best mixed with the flavors of other fruits such as strawberries, raspberries, or apples. Puree the blackcurrants and use them in foods and ice creams.

- **Blueberries.** These berries are sweet enough to eat without sweeteners. They are also good in pancakes, cakes, either lightly poached and spooned over ice cream, or baked into blueberry muffins.

- **Cherries.** Sweet varieties are good raw and can be added to salads. More bitter varieties can be used in tarts, compotes, and pancake fillings, or as a sauce for meats.

- **Plums.** Lots of varieties are available throughout summer. Most are sweet enough to eat fresh or baked. You can make them into

---

[45] Molly Watson, "Summer Fruits And Vegetables," updated Sept. 14, 2020, available at https://1ref.us/1u3, accessed 12/12/20.

crumbles, pies, or tarts. Put a few slices in green or fruit salads, or bake them alongside meat.

- **Raspberries.** Eat fresh, mix with other fruit in salads or compotes, fill flans or scones, puree to make sorbet, ice cream or a tangy sweet sauce.

- **Redcurrants.** These are charming but tart. Add to blackcurrants and stew with sugar for pies, crumbles, or summer pudding.

- **Strawberries.** The top summer fruit.

- **White currants.** See redcurrants.

## VEGETABLES

As with summer fruit, vegetables come into season in stages.

- **Asparagus.** Trim off "scales" and the tough root end, then poach, steam, or roast them with a little olive oil. Dress with vinaigrette, a little melted butter, or oil and lemon juice.

- **Aubergine (Eggplant).** There's no need to salt and drain aubergine. Rather than frying, try roasted aubergines. Slice them, brush them with oil, and then bake them in an oven until tender, then use them in casseroles and baked dishes. Ideal with tomatoes and spices.

- **Broad beans.** If you grow these beans, pick them while tiny and tender for the greatest enjoyment. Stores often carry larger pods, and the beans are less digestible. Use in salads, serve pureed, or add to soups.

- **Broccoli.** Cut broccoli into florets, eat it raw or either steam or stir-fry it briefly to preserve nutrients. It makes an excellent soup.

- **Carrots.** The smaller the sweeter. Remove leaves before storing. Eat them raw or steam, stir-fry, or roast them. A dash of orange juice brings out the taste.

- **Cauliflower.** Can be used raw in salads, steamed, or stir-fried. Cook it lightly. Mild flavor marries well with spices or vinaigrette dressing.

- **Celery.** Cut into celery sticks for snacking, chop them into salads or to add flavor to soups and stocks; you can also braise celery as an accompaniment.

- **Courgettes (Zucchini).** Young ones are the tastiest and are less watery. Slice, grate, or cut zucchini into ribbons to cook, or you can also scoop out the seeds and stuff and bake them. They can be steamed, sautéed, stir-fried, or roasted in chunks.

- **Cucumbers.** Peel and cut cucumbers into fingers for snacks; slice or chop them into salads; add diced cucumbers to bulgur wheat or couscous salads; or mix them with yogurt for a refreshing tzatziki dip.

- **French beans.** Top and tail them before steaming. Eat them hot, or let them cool off and use them in salads.

- **Globe artichoke.** The heart is the best. Remove stalks, then put artichokes in a pan of boiling water until soft enough that leaves can be removed. Then cool them and pick off the leaves and eat with dips.

- **Herbs.** Buy tender varieties—like dill, basil, and coriander—in bunches and chop them into salads, stuffing, omelets, or rice and grain dishes, or make pesto.

- **Leeks.** Keep your eye out for baby leeks to steam and serve whole. Shred or slice them to cook by steaming or stir-frying. They taste great in soups.

- **Lettuce.** There are dozens of varieties of lettuce to try throughout summer. Often it is eaten raw, but it can also be added to stir-fries or soups.

- **Mange-tout (snow peas).** Use in snow pea recipes.

- **Peas in the pod.** Peas taste best when young. Use fresh in salads or steamed. Add them to risottos, soups, or stew with a few lettuce leaves for added sweetness.

- **Peppers.** They can be red, yellow, orange, green, or even purple. Their flavor is enhanced with chargrilling, either under the grill or by baking in an oven until blistered. Put them in a plastic bag so the steam can loosen the skins and then peel and slice. Peppers are delicious raw in salads or in a stuffed pepper recipe.

- **Potatoes.** Baby potatoes are excellent in salads, or they can be steamed or roasted in their skins.

- **Radishes.** Longer, white-tipped varieties are less fiery than the red ones. They are perfect in salads or chopped into stir fries.

- **Spinach.** Choose young, tender spinach leaves. Use them raw in salads or steamed and chopped. They are great in curries with other vegetables or as a filling for savory tarts, pancakes, or omelets, or cooked in soup.

- **Swiss chard.** Its dark green leaves and red stems can be used like spinach. Its stems can also be cooked.

- **Tomatoes.** Serve fresh in salads, or in a range of tomato recipes.

- **Watercress.** The peppery flavor of watercress is good in a mixture of other leafy vegetables. It is also tasty in egg sandwiches and omelets or in soup.

Buy summer fruit and vegetables fresh every day and never suppose that you can have too much.

# CHAPTER 43

# Television[46]

Americans now spend half of their free time in front of the TV.

In a 65-year lifespan, the average person spends nine years watching television—enough time to obtain two university degrees. Children, on average, spend more time watching TV than any other activity besides sleeping.

When television is combined with video games, many teens spend 35–55 hours per week in front of the tube.

> *In a 65-year lifespan, the average person spends nine years watching television—enough time to obtain two university degrees.*

Watching TV is considered a leisure activity. Nevertheless, it leaves people passive, tense, unable to concentrate, and often in a worse mood than before watching it.

Television can also have a hypnotic, possibly addictive, and psychosocial effect. Many good programs about science, history, nature, religion, and art are available, which can stimulate interest. However, for learning, television cannot compete with books, human interaction, and real-life experience.

For every hour that preschoolers watch TV, there is a 10 percent increased risk of their having difficulty concentrating, exhibiting restlessness and impulsivity, or their being easily confused.

Television affects us mentally. Advertisers employ rapid-fire scene changes and humor to keep the viewer engaged. This reduces the ability to concentrate, which, in turn, can have negative effects on impulse control.

In response to this knowledge, you can begin a log of how much TV you're watching or how much time you spend on your phone and then begin to dial it back. One option is to fill that time by learning something new. Let self-denial and temperance be your watchword.

*Oh, that I could make all understand their obligation to God to preserve the mental and physical abilities in the best condition to render perfect service to their Maker.*

---

[46] Agata Blaszczak-Boxe, "Too Much TV Really Is Bad For Your Brain," available at https://1ref.us/1u4, accessed 12/12/20.

# CHAPTER 44

# Type 2 Diabetes[47]

Type 2 diabetes is a serious and growing malady. While age, gender, and genetics all influence risk, a healthy lifestyle can prevent and control this disease.

- Nearly 26 million people in the United States have diabetes, 7 million of whom may be undiagnosed and unaware of their condition.

- In adults 20 years of age and older, more than one in every ten people suffers from diabetes, and in seniors (aged 65 and older), that figure rises to more than one in four.

- If either parent suffers from Type 2 diabetes, a child's risk of developing the disease is 15% higher than children without a diabetic parent. If both parents have the condition, the risk of developing it is 75% higher.

- The most cost-effective prevention methods include regular physical activity and a healthy diet. Regular visits to a health care provider and maintaining a healthy weight are also essential for being able to identify risks, prevent Type 2 diabetes, and delay its onset.

- The Diabetes Prevention Program found that weight loss and increased physical activity reduced the development of Type 2 diabetes by 58%.

- Overweight individuals who lose even 5–7% of their body weight by exercising and healthy eating may effectively prevent or delay the onset of Type 2 diabetes indefinitely.

It's a good idea to obtain regular checks of blood cholesterol levels, blood pressure, and blood sugar levels to monitor your risk factors. Having healthy levels of these three indicators significantly reduces your risk of diabetes and can pay great dividends for good health.

[47] "Type 2 Diabetes: Life doesn't end with type 2 diabetes," available at https://1ref.us/1u5, accessed 12/12/20.

# CHAPTER 45

# Walnuts[48]

A handful of walnuts a day can really keep the doctor away. A new study found that eating a handful of walnuts every day may be linked to better diet quality and improvements in certain Type 2 diabetes risk factors.

Individuals who consumed walnuts every day for six months saw improvements in blood vessel function and LDL (or "bad") cholesterol levels compared to those who didn't.

Patients' BMIs (body mass indices) were found to surge on the walnut-rich diet. While walnuts contain essential fatty acids and other nutrients, they are also high in calories.

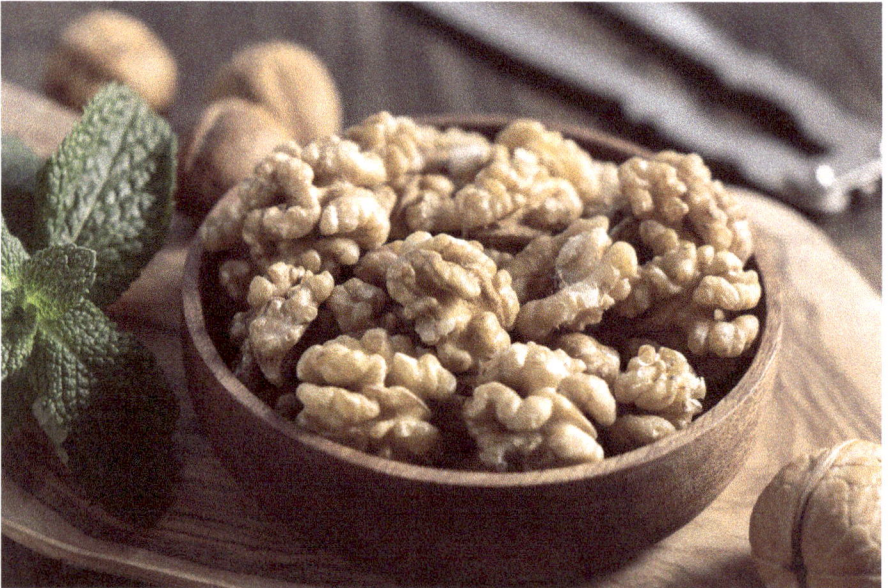

A quarter cup of walnuts, for instance, provides more than 100 percent of the daily recommended value of plant-based omega-3 fats, along with high amounts of copper, manganese, molybdenum, and biotin.

---

[48] Amanda DeWitt, "10 Surprising Benefits of Walnuts You May Not Know About," available at https://1ref.us/1u6, accessed 12/12/20.

Walnuts offer:

1.  Cancer-fighting properties
2.  Goodness for your heart
3.  Polyphenols that may prevent chemically induced liver damage
4.  Weight control and brain health benefits

The outermost layer of a shelled walnut—the whitish, flaky (or sometimes waxy) part—has a bitter flavor, but do not discard it. Up to 90 percent of the antioxidants in walnuts are found in the skin. To increase encouraging health impacts, look for *organic and raw walnuts*, not irradiated or pasteurized ones.

# CHAPTER 46

# Water for the Elderly

Two thirds of the body consists of water. However, the percentage of total body water is about 10% lower in seniors.

Older adults also have a reduced muscle mass and sometimes less functioning kidneys. They may become dehydrated without being aware of the need to increase their fluid intake.

Dehydration can cause a fever, which, undetected, increases the body's need for water.

*Older adults who are on bed rest and taking medications are at greatest risk of deydration.*

Severe dehydration puts a greater strain on the heart.

Older adults who are on bed rest and taking medications are at greatest risk of deydration. They may also fear incontinence, so they drink less fluids.[49]

Dehydration is also difficult to diagnose. Signs of dehydration in seniors may include:

| Confusion | Inability to sweat or produce tears |
|---|---|
| Difficulty walking | Rapid heart rate |
| Dizziness or headaches | Low blood pressure |
| Dry mouth | Low urine output |
| Sunken eyes | Constipation[50] |

Encourage the elderly to take small and frequent drinks of water throughout the day to maintain adequate fluids, and don't forget that fruits and vegetables are also water-laden.

*Do not cast me off in the time of old age; do not forsake me when my strength fails.* (Psalm 71:9, NKJV)

[49] Priscilla T. LeMone, Karen M. Burke, Gerene Bauldoff, and Paula Gubrud, *Medical-Surgical Nursing: Clinical Reasoning in Patient Care*, 6th ed., 2015, p. 184.
[50] Angelike Gaunt, "Dehydration in the Elderly: Signs and Prevention," June 13, 2020, available at https://1ref.us/1u7, accessed 8/10/21.

# Chapter 47

# Whole Grains[51]

Whole grains or foods made from them contain the essential and naturally occurring nutrients of the entire seed. If the grain has been processed (e.g., cracked, crushed, rolled, extruded, or cooked), the product may not deliver the same balance of nutrients found in the original, uncooked form.

100% of the original kernel—all of the bran, germ, and endosperm—must be present to qualify as a whole grain.

Here are some examples of whole grains:

- Barley
- Oats, including oatmeal
- Quinoa
- Rice, both brown rice and colored rice
- Rye
- Wheat, including varieties such as spelt, emmer, farro, einkorn, Kamut®, and durum, as well as prepared forms such as bulgur, cracked wheat, and wheatberries
- Wild rice

What is the difference between whole wheat and whole grain?

Whole wheat is one type of whole grain. Indeed, all whole wheat is a whole-grain product, but not all whole grains are whole wheat. There are whole-grain oats, whole-grain rice, etc.

Eating whole grains instead of refined grains lowers the risk of many chronic diseases. To lower that risk, we should consume at least three servings daily.

The benefits of whole grains include:

[51] Wholegrainscouncil.org, "Whole Grains 101," available at https://1ref.us/1u8, accessed 12/12/20.

- Stroke risk reduced 30–36%
- Type 2 diabetes risk reduced 21–30%
- Heart disease risk reduced 25–28%
- Better weight maintenance

Other benefits indicated by recent studies include:

- Reduced risk of asthma
- Healthier carotid arteries
- Reduced risk of inflammatory disease
- Lower risk of colorectal cancer
- Healthier blood pressure levels
- Less gum disease and tooth loss

"The earth is the Lord's, and the fullness thereof." This earth is the Lord's storehouse, from which we are ever drawing. He has provided fruits and grains and vegetables for our sustenance.

# CHAPTER **48**

# Wholesome Nutrients to Welcome Spring

We look forward to spring because it marks the end of cold weather and the emergence of the new season's bounty. Spring fruits and vegetables that are green, delicious, and unusual have unique nutritional benefits.

Consuming these foods in their immature state may mean higher levels of antioxidants and phytonutrients. Some of these foods are:

**Bee Pollen.**[52] Busy bees this time of year produce a lot of bee pollen, which has been shown to help support the immune system.

**Chia Seeds and Microgreens.**[53] These seeds yield from the chia plant, but they have a dissimilar nutritional profile. They are packed with omega-3 fatty acids, protein, and soluble fiber that the plant doesn't provide.

Tiny microgreens, such as pea shoots and broccoli sprouts, are undeveloped greens with the same vitamins (like A, C, and K) as their mature counterparts, albeit in a smaller package. Their nutrient density is more concentrated, and they have a stronger flavor.

**Wild Ramps.**[54] Ramps are a delicate shoot available in early spring. This onion counterpart is rich in vitamin A, which is essential for forming the mucous membranes of the eyes, respiratory tract, and digestive system. They act as protective barriers to keep germs at bay.

---

[52] Cathy Wong, "What Is Bee Pollen?," available at https:// https://1ref.us/1u9, accessed 12/1/20.

[53] Uyory Choe, Liangli Lucy Yu, and Thomas T. Y. Wang, "The Science behind Microgreens as an Exciting New Food for the 21st Century," available at https://1ref.us/1ua, accessed 12/1/20.

[54] Scott Sheu, "Foods Indigenous to the Western Hemisphere," available at https://1ref.us/1ub, accessed 12/1/20.

# Why *Not* to Peel These 12 Fruits and Vegetables[55]

A lot of the nutrients are discarded from our fruits by taking off the skin. Eating an entire orange may be dubious, but its peel has nearly twice as much vitamin C as the inside. Yet, there are plenty of ways to consume orange peels by getting creative. In fact, the peel is often the most nutritious.

Below are some fruits that contain nutrients in their skins.

**Apples.** The skin of an apple contains about half of the apple's overall dietary fiber content. A medium apple also delivers 9 milligrams of vitamin C, 100 IUs of vitamin A, and 200 grams of potassium. By removing the peel, about a third of those nutrients are lost. The peel also has four times more vitamin K than its flesh, about 5 percent of your daily value. Vitamin K is also prevalent in spinach and other green veggies.

**Bananas.** A banana's peel contains way more fiber than its flesh, and is likewise richer in potassium. The peel also contains lutein, a powerful antioxidant that plays a role in maintaining healthy eye function. You can blend the peel in your juicer.

**Citrus Fruits.** An orange peel packs in twice as much vitamin C as what's inside. It also contains higher concentrations of riboflavin, vitamin B6, calcium, magnesium, and potassium. The peel's flavonoids have anticancer and anti-inflammatory properties. (Citrus fruit also boosts iron absorption.) Though the peels are more challenging to digest, you can add peel shavings to salads, soups, and even desserts.

**Carrots.** The dark green skin of cucumbers contains the majority of the cucumber's antioxidants, insoluble fiber, and potassium.

**Kiwi.**

**Eggplant** skin helps protect against cancerous development.

**Mango.**

---

[55] Ann Cha and Angela Cheng Matsuzawa, "12 amazingly good and healthy uses for fruit and vegetable peel," available at https://1ref.us/1uc, accessed 12/5/20.

**Onion skins** can be added to stews and taken out prior to eating

**Pineapple.**

**Potatoes.** A potato's skin packs more nutrients—iron, calcium, potassium, magnesium, vitamin B6 and vitamin C—ounce for ounce than the rest of the potato. Ditch the skin and you lose up to 90 percent of a potato's iron content and half of its fiber. Also, the skin of a sweet potato is loaded with a significant amount of beta-carotene, which converts to vitamin A during digestion. Vitamin A is essential for cell health and immune system regulation, and it is extremely useful in maintaining organ function.

**Watermelon.**

*Grains with fruits, nuts, and vegetables, contain all the nutritive properties necessary to make good blood. (Child Guidance, p. 384)*

# Chapter 50

# Winter Fruits and Vegetables[56]

Sparkly snowflakes, cozy blankets, rich hot carob—winter has a lot going for it, but fresh produce is not often on that list. In colder climates, eating locally through the winter can be challenging. The good news is that every meal doesn't have to revolve around potatoes and onions until April. With a bit of planning and creativity, it's possible to eat fresh produce with plenty of nutrients and flavor all winter long.

Some vitamin-rich, cold-weather products of the harvest to stock up on right now are:

**Citrus fruit and Pomegranates.**

**Cabbage** is a super-healthy, budget-friendly vegetable. Cabbage is loaded with vitamins and minerals (vitamins C and K and folate, in particular), fiber, antioxidants, and anticarcinogenic compounds. It can even reduce cholesterol and lower the risk of cancer and diabetes.

**Beets.** Beets are rich in vitamins A, B, and C as well as potassium and folate.

**Brussels Sprouts,** the mini-me of cabbage, boast some of the same health benefits.

**Carrots** are loaded with the antioxidant beta-carotene.

**Onions** are ideal for flavoring anything from soup to grain, to salads, to pasta, to meat. They are low in calories but surprisingly high in vitamin C and fiber. The oils in onions can lower LDL cholesterol ("bad cholesterol") levels and raise HDL cholesterol("good cholesterol").

**Parsnips** are loaded with fiber, potassium, vitamin C, and folate. They have a slightly sweet, earthy flavor to accompany any winter soup, stew, or casserole.

**Sweet Potatoes** are loaded with fiber, beta-carotene, vitamins A and C, and antioxidants.

**Turnips and Rutabagas.**

---

[56] SNAP Education Connection, "Seasonal Produce Guide," available at https://1ref.us/1ud, accessed 12/12/20.

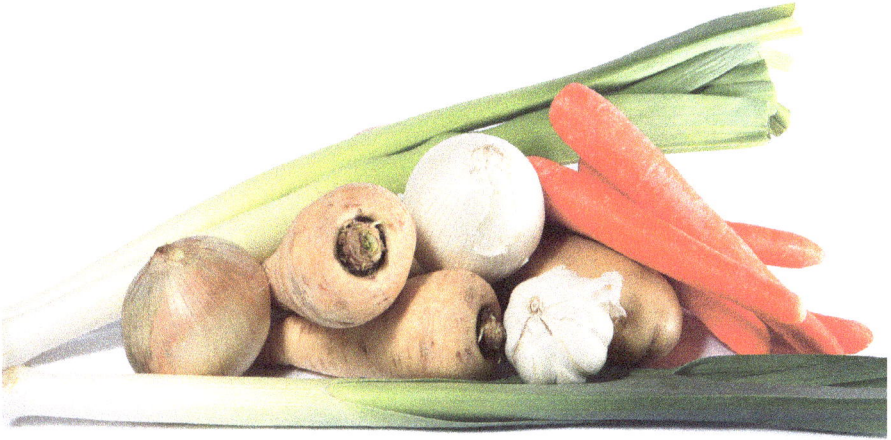

**Winter Squash.** Acorn, butternut, kabocha, and delicata squash are at their prime in the fall and winter. All are loaded with healthy goodness like carotenoids, vitamin A, and potassium.

**TEACH Services, Inc.**
P U B L I S H I N G

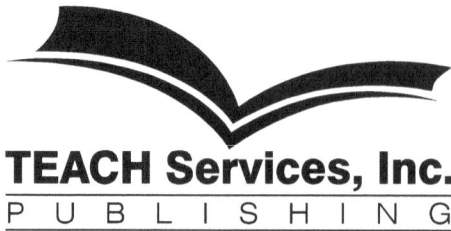

We invite you to view the complete
selection of titles we publish at:
**www.TEACHServices.com**

We encourage you to write us
with your thoughts about this,
or any other book we publish at:
**info@TEACHServices.com**

TEACH Services' titles may be purchased in
bulk quantities for educational, fund-raising,
business, or promotional use.
**bulksales@TEACHServices.com**

Finally, if you are interested in seeing
your own book in print, please contact us at:
**publishing@TEACHServices.com**
We are happy to review your manuscript at no charge.

www.ingramcontent.com/pod-product-compliance
Lightning Source LLC
Chambersburg PA
CBHW040136270326
41927CB00019B/3406